CLEANING HOUSE

CLEANING HOUSE

The Fight to Rid Our Homes of Toxic Chemicals

LINDSAY DAHL

DEYST.
An Imprint of William Morrow

DEYST.

This book was written from memory spanning the course of twenty years, and while my memory is sharp, like anyone's it is imperfect. I've done my best to be faithful to my lived experiences and where possible consulted others who were present during that time. In addition, I relied on documents, journals, live interviews, and conversations I had with many people who appear in these pages. In some cases, I have edited conversations for brevity and storytelling or truthfully recalled them from memory when transcripts were not available. To protect the anonymity of certain individuals, I have modified their identifying details and/or their names. The content presented is based on my perspective and does not reflect the views or opinions of past, present, or future employers.

FIRST EDITION

Library of Congress Cataloging-in-Publication Data has been applied for.

ISBN 978-0-06-337559-8

25 26 27 28 29 LBC 5 4 3 2 1

To my daughters:
I love you no matter what.

In Memory Of

Leaders Whose Lives Ended Too Soon
Fernando (Andy) Igrejas, 1970–2018
Cecil Corbin Mark, 1969–2020

Legislative Champions Who Led the Fight
Senator Frank Lautenberg, 1924–2013
Author and champion of the Lautenberg Chemical Safety Act

Senator Diane Feinstein, 1933–2023
Lead author and champion of the Safe Cosmetics Act

CONTENTS

An Important Note to Readers

If there's one thing I know to be true from my years of lobbying and grassroots organizing, it's that people remember stories, especially those about people, more than they remember facts. So I am telling the story of the environmental health movement through the lens of my own experience and through the stories of experts I've crossed paths with over the years. I have chosen several leaders to feature and I'm deeply grateful for the time they spent with me for the book. Please know that these experts are a small selection of a large movement of thousands of scientists, business leaders, elected officials, social justice organizers, and many more people who have contributed to our progress to remove toxic chemicals from our environment, communities, and bodies.

My hope is that you learn along with me over my career, laughing at my many missteps and grappling with the same shocking discoveries I faced. Ultimately, I hope you land where I did: clear-eyed and resolved to help make a difference. The movement to rid our world of poisons is made up of thousands of leaders who have all contributed in meaningful ways.

Over the course of these pages, I unpack the science, politics, and culture of "clean" as a foundation for joining and engaging in this movement in the highest-impact way. Perhaps most important, there is a comprehensive Take Action section at the end that gives you clear, science-backed tips for shopping the market for safer products, non-partisan ways to help pass new chemical safety laws, and honest questions to ask yourself on how we collectively shape the culture behind this important movement. I hope that by the end of the book, you will join us.

INTRODUCTION

I LIFT MY THREE-YEAR-OLD DAUGHTER INTO THE BAS-
ket of a bright red Target cart and let her older sister ride on the
side. Bringing along two young children means it will inevitably
be a stressful shopping trip (one that would take eight minutes if I
were solo), so I've prepared: I have a short list of must-get items in
my right hand and responses ready for their inevitable requests for
flashy toys. Pulling into aisle B20, I look at a wall of water bottles
and from the cart I hear, "Mom, can we get that Moana water
bottle?!" "Go that way, I see stuffies!" I try to tune out their shouts
and take a moment to reflect on the marketing language on nearly
every plastic water bottle on the shelf: "BPA-free." I smile, happy
to see how easy it is for shoppers to ID a water bottle without this
particular toxic chemical.

Twenty years earlier, when I started working on consumer safety
issues as a lobbyist for an environmental health nonprofit, I was
part of the early crew working to educate lawmakers on the dangers
of chemicals like bisphenol A (BPA). And it is bad: BPA is an endocrine disruptor that can mess with our hormones, especially during
vulnerable windows of development like childhood. Back then,
eyes would glaze over when I rattled off names of toxic chemicals

like BPA, phthalates, flame retardants, and VOCs. Today you can't find a single baby bottle on the shelves that contains BPA. I opt for a stainless steel water bottle, knowing it'll be safer for my girls, and thankfully there are some fun bright colors they can choose from to compete with Moana.

From here on out, I'm on autopilot. The remainder of the trip is a succession of similarly quick, informed decision-making: in the personal care aisle I grab a bar of soap from a trusted brand formulated without the worst chemical offenders, bypassing the big-name household companies that announce "nature-made" on the label despite being fragranced with undisclosed ingredients. It's a move known as "greenwashing"—when companies use language and packaging to make a product seem eco-friendly and to signal safety. The fact is that these terms aren't regulated at all. "Nature-made" or "nontoxic" or "clean" doesn't mean that any criteria were met for quality or safety—it's simply language that makes the customer think that the product is harmless and good for them.

In the shoe aisle, a row of children's rain boots dazzle in front of me. My oldest starts wiggling to show me she needs to use the restroom ASAP, so I quickly grab the garden-themed rubber boots instead of the sparkly pink vinyl ones. I know that rubber is the obvious choice: Vinyl is nicknamed the "poison plastic" because it can release carcinogens and phthalates from manufacture to disposal, poisoning communities and people using the products in their home.

In the children's toy section, I let each daughter pick one Paw Patrol figurine. I choose these, as they're typically made from a plastic called ABS, and while far from my top choice of materials, it has a much lower risk of leaching toxic chemicals compared to other plastics. I can't be 100 percent certain it's ABS, since there are no material labeling requirements for many product categories, including children's toys. Still, in this moment, I'm okay with the gamble, based on the risk matrix in my head. While I take meaningful steps to protect my kids, I also don't want to be that mom, the inflexible one who says "no" constantly, is afraid of everything, and sucks the spontaneity out of life. Skye and Marshall are coming home, and my kids are pumped.

This is how I move through the world: balancing the reality that I can't control everything with a deep understanding of how the everyday items I bring into my home and expose my family to, matter for us, for the workers making the products, and for the planet and the population at large. It's a high-wire act.

We make a pit stop at the restroom, and then I load my kids into my minivan (I'm cool, don't worry). I'm exhausted. It's hard taking two kids under five to Target while navigating a complex marketplace. And I have a privilege that most do not: I have a 360-degree view into the life cycle of most consumer products. With that knowledge, I can balance my finances so that, for the riskiest product categories, I can opt into purchasing safer brands, which in some cases are pricier.

But even with that knowledge, the whole scenario makes me sad. And angry.

No consumer should need a degree in chemistry or spend hours doing online research (or have a friend like me in their phone) to win the game of "spot the toxic ingredient" as they shop. It really shouldn't be this hard to protect ourselves from toxic chemicals. In fact, it isn't this hard in other countries, where they have taken a more proactive approach to removing toxic chemicals from products.

I brood over all of this as I head to the gas station, one last stop before home. It's ironic, but the process of filling up our gas tanks is far simpler and arguably safer than a trip to a big-box store. We don't have to research how dangerous it might be to inhale lead fumes at the pump, or suss out which locations sell lead-free gas. We don't have to decipher marketing jargon to determine whether or not the heavy metal is lurking in a list of additives. That's because, in 1996, the Environmental Protection Agency (EPA)—thanks to a mountain of science showing that inhaling leaded gasoline fumes is linked to lower IQ, seizures, and irreversible brain damage— barred the heavy metal from being added to gas via the national Clean Air Act. While I'm in no way saying that gasoline is "clean," this major piece of public health protection (along with banning lead from household paint) has resulted in a 90 percent drop in the lead levels of Americans' bodies over a nineteen-year period. None of us notice how much safer we are at a gas station today compared to thirty years ago. When public health regulations are working, they're often invisible.

And that is the kind of protection we deserve at every point of sale, not just at the pump. Part of the challenge is the inconspicuous nature of many toxic chemicals. Inhaling leaded-gasoline fumes? Sure, that clocks as harmful. But who would think the cute vinyl rain boots can cause serious health issues for children? I mean, they're covered in flowers.

Here's the shocking truth: the science showing how poisonous the chemicals in our consumer products are is as strong as the science that led the government to ban lead from gasoline and place warnings about cancer on cigarette packs. These days we accept that "smoking causes lung cancer," "lead is toxic," and "asbestos can kill you" because we've been living with these evidence-based truths for decades, and thankfully, there are some regulations in place protecting us. But the impact of other chemicals, ones that keep environmental health scientists up at night and have the same level of rock-solid backing as the dangers of asbestos and lead, are being ignored—by the people we elect to protect us and by the corporations that create the chemicals in the first place and profit off of them.

And off of us.

The idea that we're in real danger from everyday household items is sobering and perhaps even questionable for people who haven't gotten a peek under the hood. If you come to this book with a discerning eye, we have that in common. I started out as a skeptic. It's my nature to not take anything for granted, and I have a tendency to annoy friends and colleagues by taking a contrarian position to most things right off the bat. I rolled my eyes when, twenty years ago, an activist told me that my household dust was toxic. I questioned the science when a friend warned that my lip gloss was hacking my hormones, thinking she'd fallen prey to a conspiracy theory.

A lot has changed for me over the past two decades. I read the studies and interviewed the scientists, some of whom you will meet in the pages of this book, people who have been doing groundbreaking research linking toxic chemicals to an array of conditions: cancer, asthma, birth defects, immune system damage, and infertility, marked by a 50 percent global drop in sperm counts over the last fifty years. That statistic sounds unbelievable, but nothing I will share in this book is overstated—I'm as allergic to hyperbole and overstated science as I am to goldenrods in the fall. And know that scientists are specifically trained not to jump to conclusions. (If anything, they tend to be extra cautious.) I've met firefighters who have experienced the devastating health effects of breathing in the toxic flame retardants that industry adds to furniture. And I've learned firsthand from those living close to chemical and plastic manufacturing, communities with unprecedented rates of cancers linked to toxic chemicals. I've gone up against chemical industry lobbyists and spin doctors at legislative hearings.

To state the obvious, I'm no longer a skeptic.

So why is the science there but the regulations aren't? Why are we as consumers burdened with brushing up on chemistry lessons between work meetings and doctor appointments when scientists and lawmakers know better? Why do we all know the details of the latest celebrity scandal, but not how the ingredients in a best-selling body lotion can easily damage our reproductive systems?

Three major things are keeping us stuck in our toxic world. All are fixable—that's why I wrote this book—but until we understand these fundamental truths, we won't be able to make the changes we need to clean things up.

1. **There is a war happening between old and new science.** Representing Team Old Science is the field of toxicology, the original field of science meant to help us understand how much of a certain poison will hurt or kill us. (And by "old science" I mean old—we're talking the sixteenth century, just before microscopes were invented.) Old science is somewhat helpful when trying to determine, say, how much extra-strength Tylenol will harm your child. (I speak from experience—it looked like candy apparently, and thankfully my kids are fine.) But it's not very helpful in determining how microscopic toxic chemicals damage our delicate body systems. Chemical companies love old science, and they want you to love it too. Their greatest hits include "Cigarettes aren't that bad—just ask Joe Camel!" and "Formaldehyde in hair products is perfectly fiiiiine."

Team New Science—brought to you by the fields of epidemiology, oncology, endocrinology, epigenetics, biochemistry, and many others—tells us how invisible chemicals in our homes and products and air and water behave in ways we had never expected them to, hacking our endocrine and immune systems by unlocking doors that should remain shut and locking ones that we need to stay open. New science clearly shows that in some cases lower-level chronic exposures to toxic chemicals can lead to major health harms, especially during vulnerable windows such as pregnancy and childhood.

2. **The things we bring into our homes and put on our bodies are getting the least amount of scrutiny in Washington.** There are several obvious reasons for this—money, corporate greed, chemical industry influence, a growing anti-government sentiment among the American public—but some of it has to do with the war between new and old science. When politicians side with the chemical industry and old science, nothing changes. When lawmakers let companies police themselves, trusting that they will "do the right thing" on their own, we've seen time and again that corporations prioritize profits over public safety. In the instances where lawmakers have followed new science—when they've acted on the latest research and listened to consumer rights groups and medical organizations—our government has worked the way it's supposed to: protecting us by placing guardrails around how companies do business. And know that it isn't always less profitable for companies to do business in safer ways— sometimes it's more so. The explosion in the clean market and the record profits of companies that are creating safer products is proof of that.

3. **Social media is making things *way* worse.** The fact that anyone can be an "expert" is further muddying the science, making it even harder for consumers to tell what's safe. And when we're confused and overwhelmed, we're less compelled to push elected officials for better laws. The same chemical industry lies I've heard over the years defending toxic chemicals' safety—"chemical hair straighteners aren't harmful" or "we already have strong safety regulations in place"—are the very ones I'm now seeing popular TikTokers and old-school cosmetic chemists with millions of followers reel off. I also see the other extreme, the "all chemicals are bad!" brigade, pushing back with equally faulty information and scaring folks into no longer wearing sunscreen or avoiding anything with preservatives.

Social media is also making the clean living movement—the lifestyle of adopting a safer and healthier approach to eating, beauty, and cleaning—its own worst enemy. Who do you think of when someone says "clean living"? Maybe the term calls to mind the off-the-grid homeschooler who dismisses anything made in a lab and believes the government is out to get her via "chemtrails." For others, "clean living" may conjure an image of the perfectly coiffed influencer in her gleaming kitchen, where she makes cacao-avocado smoothies served in mason jars while wearing a $500 organic hemp caftan, holding up a perfectionist ideal that even she isn't meeting (no one can) when the cameras are off. These two women, while often politically and culturally on the opposite ends of the spectrum, have something in common: they are both selling a version of clean that doesn't always line up with science.

If reading this triggered you or you saw yourself in these descriptions, stay with me. Everyone is welcome and needed. By eroding our resilience, social media has made us less able to connect with people who have different political views than ourselves. But even worse, we've become so fragile that even reading something that feels like a critique of our lifestyles or political parties, makes us shut down. When this happens, the chemical industry wins.

We have made some progress that should give you hope as you read this book, but some of the laws we've already passed are in jeopardy of being undone. And so much more has to happen. We're only halfway to the finish line. Take those BPA-free water bottles at Target: they can be made using BPS (bisphenol S), a chemical cousin of BPA with similarly problematic health effects. (That's why I went for the stainless steel one.) These "regrettable substitutions" have flooded the marketplace because our laws generally don't ban an entire class of chemicals, but rather only one specific chemical for one specific product. You can see how easy it is for the chemical industry to concoct new chemicals to evade a ban, resulting in Whac-a-Mole for those of us working to clean up the marketplace and a game of Russian roulette for you. There are still major gaps in regulations; some of the most toxic chemicals are still used in products today, despite major legislative wins over the last two decades.

TL;DR, we've got a huge mess to clean up.

Wherever you sit on the spectrum from "Let's do this!" (welcome, fellow activists!) to "We're so f'd it doesn't matter" (I see you too), there is a place for you in our exit strategy—and no, you don't have to run for office or replace your entire stash of toiletries.

The most important intel I have to share with you in this book isn't which lotions get the green light or which toy you should toss out or which company to boycott (though I do include science-backed shopping tips at the end of the book). It's information on how we can fix, once and for all, these overarching problems that allow toxic chemicals to enter our products, homes, children's bodies, the air we breathe, and the water we drink in the first place.

Between the extremes of becoming a conspiracy theorist or throwing in the towel because it's just so overwhelming or complex, there's a sane middle ground that's gone missing, and that sweet spot is our best hope. Frankly, black-and-white thinking is its own public health hazard. It feeds into the stark cultural and political divides we've seen widening over the last decade and forces people to take sides with issues that shouldn't even have sides. Science— facts shouldn't have anything to do with party affiliation, but the question of whether a shampoo or baby bottle or lipstick is safe or not has become locked in a tug-of-war between the left and the right.

The way forward: we all move away from the extremes and toward the middle. Here, we follow actual science, not fearmongering or industry spin. We all want and deserve to live in a world where the products we use have met a high bar of safety, where our air and water and soil aren't delivery systems for proven poisons. We can also agree that our elected officials, whom we hired to protect us, should take steps to safeguard public health and the environment. Safer options exist—some companies are stepping up and doing the right thing—but these alternatives shouldn't be so damn hard to find and they shouldn't be so expensive, tucked away in some niche store or shoved aside by a brand using unregulated marketing lingo like "nontoxic."

What we need, and what I am offering, is a holistic, common-sense approach to tackling the root issues that are making us and our planet sick. That's the polite way of putting it. Another way to say it: let's turn this shit off at the tap so we can get on with the business of enjoying life.

Why should you trust me? I've helped pass over thirty consumer safety laws throughout my career. (See, Mom, there are good lobbyists!) In addition to being the lead strategist for the nation's first state ban on BPA in Minnesota, I managed a national grassroots movement that led to the passage of federal toxic chemical reforms that hadn't progressed since 1976. I've been at the center of nearly every piece of state and federal clean beauty legislation passed in recent years.

I've also developed and manufactured clean products through my roles at Beautycounter, a clean cosmetics company, and Ritual, a science-backed vitamin brand with a traceable supply chain. I understand what it takes for companies to make safe products. (It's way harder than it looks.) And I know that leaving it up to companies to do the right thing isn't the answer, there are limits to how "clean" a brand can make its products. The free market has had its chance to fix the problem, and it's not working. You can't shop or formulate your way out of this.

Perhaps most importantly, I'm just like anyone else: trying to find a happy medium. I'm not perfect and I don't expect anyone else to be. I've had friends tell me they're scared to invite me into their homes because they use plastic dishware and their mattresses aren't organic. I smile and reassure them: "Same." If I invited you over, you would find plastic and junk food in my cabinets. Honestly, I'm 1,000 percent okay with these choices because perfectionism is part of what's wrong with today's approach. Perfect really can be the enemy of good. The pursuit of perfection is futile and can make you want to give up altogether. So I'm good with good.

If you are feeling overwhelmed by the enormity of all the problems we face living in today's world—climate change, political standoffs, contentious family gatherings, rampant misinformation everywhere you look—and are this close to giving in to apathy, please don't. The solutions I lay out in this book actually overlap with the fixes for climate change and the polarization that is driving us apart. It's all connected. And we need you. That's not to say that any one person should feel burdened with solving this on their own—that's a trap, it truly takes a village. But the worst thing we can do is throw up our hands because it feels too all-consuming to tackle. It's not, I promise.

Some of the facts and cultural dynamics I cover in this book might make you uncomfortable—they are designed to. We all have assumptions that need to be reconsidered, including me. Ultimately, I want you to know what I know, to be privy to the jaw-dropping discoveries that I and others in the environmental health and consumer safety movement have had. I want you to understand who the real enemies are (sometimes it's painfully obvious, other times not so much), how clever and callous and selfish they can be, and how to outsmart them. I also want you to know who the good folks are, the everyday heroes you likely have never heard of. These are the people who are impacting your life, right now, in positive ways. I am telling the true and incredible tale of consumer safety so we can write the happy ending together.

The ultimate goal is to remove toxic chemicals at the source so that we don't have to consult "safe" shopping lists or try to decipher whether the latest news headline is fearmongering or legit science. Your time and energy are too precious to spend on that. You shouldn't have to worry about which lip gloss has ingredients linked to infertility or which rain boots are safest for your kid. You should be putting on that gloss before going to dinner with friends, or spending that time splashing in puddles with your kids. I know I will.

But first, I'm asking you to spend a little time on this issue now so that in a few years we don't have to.

1

THE SCIENTIST

SITTING IN MY CAR IN THE DARK UNDERGROUND PARK-
ing lot, I struggled to quickly change out of my waitress uniform
into a "work outfit" for my first important meeting. It was 2006
and I was just several months into my dream job—lobbying for
a small environmental nonprofit based in Minneapolis—and had
been invited to meet with an influential organization to learn about
a new campaign. It felt like a big deal to be asked to join—in order
to reach out, someone had to know I existed. And at twenty-two,
getting people to know you exist is the main goal.

To mask the smell of restaurant baked into my hair, I doused
myself in Bonne Bell musk perfume. I didn't know what exactly
the meeting was about, but I definitely didn't want these bigwigs
knowing I needed a second job waiting tables to make ends meet.

Little did I know that the perfume and the ingredients used to
make it would be the topic of conversation.

The hallway of their offices was dimly lit, run-down, and
musty—a vibe I'd learned was typical of nonprofits, as there wasn't

a lot of money for decor. I was greeted by a small woman in a big patchwork sweater. That wouldn't have been strange except it was the middle of summer and the air conditioning wasn't on. "Lindsay, I'm so happy you're here! I am really excited to get your organization caught up on what is happening on the front lines of environmental health science." I was immediately bored. Having majored in political science and environmental studies, I thought I had a good grasp on environmental health: lead paint is toxic, asbestos can kill you, and air pollution is linked to asthma. That was the whole story, right?

But she pushed on. "Did you hear about how CNN's Anderson Cooper was tested for toxic chemicals in his body?" No, I hadn't. I was more of a *Grey's Anatomy* viewer.

She went on to explain that apparently they'd discovered high levels of phthalates in Cooper's blood. Phthalates, the woman explained, are hormone-disrupting chemicals found in a variety of consumer goods, including personal care products. "And they linked the phthalates to the makeup he wears every night for his broadcast," she said breathlessly, before adding quietly, "Oh, and by the way, phthalates can hurt a person's ability to have a baby later in life."

This didn't sound good, but she was talking to the wrong person. In fact, I wasn't sure I wanted to be a parent. At that stage in my life, I was very actively trying not to get pregnant. Chemicals that could damage fertility and a developing fetus sounded awful, but they had little to do with my primary passion: addressing climate change.

This wasn't just about makeup and fertility, she added. Perfume also contained phthalates. I immediately regretted that Bonne Bell dousing, worried she was judging me. Kids' toys like rubber duckies also contain these chemicals and can mess with growing bodies' hormones. They can even concentrate in household dust. She finally came to the reason she'd asked me there: she wanted me to educate and rally college students, asking them to contact their legislators in support of a proposed ban on these chemicals in children's toys.

It all sounded overblown to me. Sure, there was the small part of me regretting that hefty dose of perfume, wondering if the chemicals were slowly leaching into my bloodstream, but the bigger part of me thought: How much could microscopic amounts of chemicals I'd never heard of from cosmetics, plastic cups, or even the dust in our homes really hurt us? And surely there were laws that prevented toxic chemicals from being in products we used in our homes, right?

I was also disappointed that this meeting was not about climate change. This was a "consumer safety" issue. Consumer safety made me think about seat belts and that wasn't nearly as cool as stopping the world from bursting into flames. I was fresh out of college, ready to make real change, and I wanted to be tackling the sexy issues. I also didn't see the connection to environmental causes or how I would get college students to care. Still, I was looking for another legislative issue to keep me busy and impress my new boss, so I smiled kindly as she handed me the rubber ducky–covered fact sheet, printed on yellow paper, and told her I'd look into it.

And I did. I'm skeptical by nature and always need to make sure my eye rolls are warranted. Despite it being the end of the workday, I drove back to the office. Working late hours was the only way to keep my two-job lifestyle afloat. Heading down the highway, I had no idea that what awaited me on the other side of my keyboard that night would completely pivot my career and introduce me to a world I hadn't learned anything about in my undergraduate classes: science showing alarming links between toxic chemicals in our products and the health of our bodies and the environment. A modern-day David and Goliath battle, with the chemical industry in the role of Goliath and everyday families and scientists as Davids. I was about to dive, naively, into a political landscape where dirty tricks that seemed made for the movies were happening in real life. My initial skepticism would be turned on its head, and I'd be forced to change my perspective on issues related to safety and health for decades to come.

This may all sound rather dramatic, but looking back, I can clearly see this was my first big before-and-after moment. There would be many more "oh shit" moments to follow, epiphanies revealing that what I thought I knew about the world, about chemicals and politicians and companies and even human nature, was wrong or vastly different than what I expected. Some of my discoveries would leave me heartsick and angry and scared for the future; in other instances, I would be blown away by the intelligence, resilience, and goodness of people working toward a safer world, often on behalf of those with the least agency—babies, pregnant women, vulnerable communities. And through it all, I learned that systems we've been conditioned to trust—the marketplace, the legislative process, social media—are complicated at best and downright inept or contaminated at worst. But I also learned that our collective voices and active participation in those very systems can course-correct just about anything.

Arriving at the office, long after everyone had left, I put Radiohead on my iPod and searched "scientific studies on the health effects of BPA and phthalates." I sat in front of the glow of the giant turquoise Apple monitor as the results populated. What Google delivered was concerning. I scrolled through the results carefully, ignoring anything that wasn't peer-reviewed, the gold standard of research, meaning a study that has been scrutinized by experts in the field. I was shocked by what I found. Study after study from top-tier journals showcased how phthalates and BPA disrupted the normal functioning of hormone systems and in turn fertility and fetal development. I read abstracts (the top-line findings) explaining that teething toys and baby bottles could leach BPA and phthalates and that the chemicals were also being detected in wildlife.

Shit. The woman in the big sweater was right.

As I dug deeper, I traced the origin of these chemicals back to an entity I knew well from my studies on climate pollution: the fossil fuel industry. All these chemicals were made from petroleum. Consumer safety had suddenly become a sexier—and far more urgent—issue.

I called my roommates to let them know I was going to miss happy hour. I wanted to zoom in and understand how these chemicals were playing out inside our bodies. The ways they worked seemed counter to what I had learned in school: "the dose makes the poison," meaning, if it's just a little bit, it can't hurt you. Surely, I thought, a bigger dose was more dangerous.

What I learned was fascinating and horrifying. Microscopic amounts of toxic chemicals from household products were apparently acting like natural hormones, turning on and off all sorts of signals that govern major body systems—the reproductive system, metabolism, and even some brain function. Hormones are like keys that open locked doors, and thanks to thousands of years of evolution, they are finely tuned to open certain doors at certain times so we can hit puberty at the right time, grow a healthy baby, and so on. The problem is that our bodies don't know the difference between natural hormones (created by our bodies) and synthetic ones (like the BPA in a baby bottle). Phthalates and BPA were scrambling the signals, opening doors that should have stayed locked and locking ones that should have been open. It was like giving a set of master keys to a monkey. I felt I was reading the script of a sci-fi thriller in which synthetic hormones played the role of invisible intruders and our bodies were the unsuspecting victims.

As I sat at my desk reading studies about phthalates, one woman's name kept coming up more than any other: Shanna Swan, PhD, a reproductive health researcher at the Icahn School of Medicine at Mount Sinai in New York. Swan was the lead author of a new study that had been widely picked up in the mainstream press, which was unusual for news about a chemical with a hard-to-pronounce name. Swan and her team had shown that pregnant women whose urine contained the highest concentrations of four specific phthalate metabolites (the term for the chemicals after they have been metabolized by the body) also had the highest chance of giving birth to boys with smaller genitals. This condition included a shorter distance between the anus and the genitals—known as anogenital distance (AGD)—as well as a smaller penis and an increased chance of undescended testicles. I discovered with a few more clicks why these things mattered so much: undescended testicles are linked to lower sperm counts, fertility issues, and testicular cancer in animal studies. Apparently, Swan's study had answered a question that scientists around the world had been asking: Were phthalates found in our home environments—in shampoo and perfume and toys and plastics—linked to changes in humans? The answer was clear: yes, they were. And we knew enough not to put them in children's toys, baby bottles, or sippy cups.

I stared at my computer, stunned. Why hadn't I heard about any of this? Sure I was young, but I considered myself to be savvy, and here was a massive body of science unfolding that I didn't know a thing about. I was surprised that none of my college instructors had even alluded to this new understanding of how toxic chemicals behave in our bodies, given that our lives were permeated with them. I started thinking about the various plastic cups in my kitchen (made durable from BPA), the plastic toy I had just bought for my niece (made flexible by the addition of phthalates), the makeup and scented lotion I slathered on my dry legs, and the fragranced laundry detergent I washed my clothes with. (Scent, I'd learned, was bound to skin and clothing thanks to certain phthalates.)

One thing I read was particularly bugging me. The European Union (EU) had recently banned fourteen hundred chemicals in personal care products—compared to the meager eleven restricted in the United States. So companies based in the States were already making two different versions of their shampoos, lotions, and mascaras—one to sell domestically and one to sell in European countries with stricter laws. Manufacturers had clearly figured out how to make good-smelling lotion and shampoo for Europeans without using these chemicals. But they weren't bothering to sell those safer versions here.

The double standard was exactly the kind of thing I knew I could get college students to care about, mostly because it pissed me off. I asked the internet one last question for the night: "Has the EU banned phthalates?" Answer: yes. The EU had banned the use of two phthalates—DEHP and DBP—from cosmetics in 2004. I cross-referenced those with the phthalates that Swan had studied and the ones Sweater Woman wanted us to help ban.

They were one and the same.

Over the next few days, fired up but still a little skeptical—and incredulous—I dug deeper into the research and health effects of phthalates. I wasn't the only one meeting the topic with a critical eye, as it turned out. Shanna Swan also started out as a skeptic. Years later, she'd share with me how her career arc shifted when she discovered these alarming trends. She is efficient with her time and expects you to be as well. It's almost like you can feel the clock ticking, knowing we have little time to act before permanently altering the future of human reproduction. It sounds dramatic, but it's also true. Swan is quite measured in her presentation of how chemicals from everyday products are hacking our natural systems in ways we don't want them to. She stays in the knowledge lane, never veering into unproven suppositions.

Swan didn't start out studying phthalates—she happened upon them. Working for Kaiser Permanente in the early 1990s, she had her first run-in with the effects of hormones on human health. One of her areas of research was studying possible links between estrogen in birth control pills, sexual activity, and cervical cancer. "It's not obvious, but oral contraceptives are hormone disruptors. That's why we take them, right?" she asked rhetorically on one of our calls. As a statistician, she was looking at large and complicated datasets, work she describes as tedious but also satisfying in a cut-and-dried way. The numbers were stripped of bias; analyzing Excel spreadsheets was a matter of fact, not opinion.

By 1995, having started to make a name for herself as a powerhouse statistician in the field of endocrinology, Swan was invited to sit on a committee of the National Academy of Sciences examining the impact of hormonally active agents in the environment. She was honored by the invitation—the committee members were among the loftiest in the scientific research universe—but when she joined the committee she was undecided, even skeptical, about the role of "accidental" (unintentional) exposures to endocrine disruptors (hormone-mimicking chemicals) through environmental routes, such as the air or skin or the water supply. It was a fairly little known topic at the time, even for Swan, who hadn't heard the term "endocrine-disrupting chemical" before. As the only statistician on the panel, she was tasked with examining the data behind a well-known Danish study that found an alarming decline in sperm counts. Was the sharp decline in sperm counts the scientists reported real?

She herself questioned whether the dramatic numbers—a 50 percent drop over fifty years—were real. In fact, no one on the committee, including Swan, was convinced that the study was solid. But intrigued, she agreed to take a look. She figured that she'd spot an issue with the data collecting, or discover that some men had confounding factors—such as stress or obesity—that would explain the drop. Swan spent six months looking at the question. "The results turned my life around," she told me.

Swan reworked the data from the sixty-one studies and even added forty more studies to pressure-test the numbers. She deconstructed the studies, separating out factors like threads on separate spools, then stitching them back together in various ways to reveal any loose ends. After multiple attempts, nothing changed. The conclusion was the same every time: sperm counts had plummeted.

Swan went back to the committee and reported, "This is real. There has been a decline in sperm count. But we don't know why." In 1997, the results of her analysis put "environmental endocrine disrupting agents" and sperm decline on the map. The problem: there wasn't yet a smoking gun linking hormone disruption to declining sperm counts—or to other health issues raised in the report, such as breast cancer. Researchers had articulated the what but not the why. Swan remained open to what was causing the sperm count decline, as scientists are trained to do when they don't have data tipping them in one direction or another. She reached out to a few geneticists, asking: Was it a gene mutation?

No, the timetable was too fast for these changes to show up in a generation or two. It had to be something else.

It wasn't until a few years later, when Swan was 30,000 feet above the Pacific on her way to Japan to present findings at a conference, that she serendipitously learned about research that would lead her to that smoking gun. She was traveling with John Brock, a Centers for Disease Control and Prevention (CDC) chemist heading to the same meeting. When neither immediately cracked open their airplane book, they started talking, swapping information about their research. Brock shared that the CDC was measuring something called phthalates in the urine of women who were participants in the NHANES (National Health and Nutrition Examination Survey) study, a huge, ongoing research program. "You should study phthalates," he told her. "Why?" she asked. She'd never heard of them. Brock explained how phthalates were used across a variety of products found in our homes, from added fragrance in deodorants and hair products to making plastic containers soft, and that studies had shown alarming health trends in rats—phthalate exposure in pregnant rats disrupted the genital development of their male babies in utero by affecting their testosterone levels. The male mice were born with shorter penises, sometimes deformed penises, undescended testicles, and shorter anogenital distance (or, in common slang, "taint").

Swan was fascinated. "We're finding that nearly everyone has some level of phthalates in their body," he explained. For hours on the long flight, Swan soaked up the details, and by the time the plane landed in Tokyo she was buzzing with the implications.

Right away, Swan began digging into the data about how the chemicals dampen testosterone in the body and reached out to the person who'd done the seminal research on rats. Paul Foster had discovered that the exposed male offspring were not completely masculinized, that when testosterone was hijacked by phthalates, it couldn't complete its mission. Not only that, but there was a really specific window in the gestation of rats—day 18 to day 21—when phthalate exposure would send baby rats on a developmentally altered course.

Swan was ready to examine whether something similar was occurring in humans. Luckily, she had collected and stored urine samples from pregnant mothers several years earlier for the study she had presented in Japan that looked at whether exposure from certain pesticides affected sperm quality in men. (Spoiler alert: it does.) She didn't know why she was collecting the pregnant partners' urine at the time; she just figured it was easy and they had access to a freezer. (Who among us hasn't stored human urine in the freezer just in case?) Her curiosity paid off. Most mothers from the study agreed to be recontacted, and by now, three years later, their babies had been born.

Swan got to work studying the boys born to those pregnant mothers from her earlier study, measuring AGD along with penis length, testicular volume, and the placement of testicles. After evaluating the data, she had her answer: higher levels of phthalate metabolites in a pregnant mom's urine were strongly associated with a baby boy's risk of having a short AGD, a shorter penis, and undescended testicles—the same phthalates Dr. Brock had referenced on the plane ride to Japan. This was the study I'd stumbled upon and was about to give me ammunition to lobby that "small doses" of these chemicals were unsafe.

Seven years later, in 2011, Swan published another pivotal study showing that phthalate syndrome and a short AGD were associated with a significant harm in human males: lower sperm counts. Further studies would reveal a greater risk of brain development problems in both males and females born to moms with high phthalate exposure. These harms included lower IQ and a reduction in gray matter, the brain tissue used for all-important processes like controlling muscles and retaining information. In 2017, Swan led the largest analysis of sperm count trends, dissecting data from over 42,000 men reported in more than 2,500 scientific articles. The data and methodology were bulletproof: over a forty-year time span, they found a 50 to 60 percent decline in sperm counts worldwide.

This was the moment it all clicked for Swan: phthalates were the missing link.

My own "oh shit" moment, sparked by Swan's 2005 study, was a turning point for my career. Up until that fateful day, I'd been focused on lobbying for climate change, but just like that, my focus became environmental health. (I would later understand that the two are deeply connected.) Something in me had shifted. When I opened my kitchen cabinet or bathroom vanity, lifted the lid of my laundry machine, or pulled back my vinyl shower curtain, I kept asking myself the same question: "Can I trust that this is safe?"

The answer, every time, was no.

If that wasn't infuriating enough, I couldn't believe that the burden of ascertaining safety rested on the shoulders of consumers. Why should I have to become a chemist and decipher what was safe and unsafe on store shelves? I had enough to worry about between working two jobs, staying fed, and trying to have a social life. Why wasn't this the responsibility of the companies making the chemicals and products we brought into our homes, or the government agencies that existed to manage oversight? If something was harmful, shouldn't it just be removed from the market altogether?

And even though I had no interest in becoming a mother at that point, what scared me was how these chemicals impacted the most vulnerable among us: babies. Some of my closest relatives were getting ready to start their own families, and surely they didn't have this information either. If I were trying to get pregnant, how would I know exactly when to eliminate exposures to phthalates? Was there a time when the fetus was most vulnerable? One of Swan's later studies would estimate that the key window of susceptibility for reproductive harms during human gestation is between eight and fourteen weeks. And it's pretty common not to know you're pregnant at eight weeks (as I would later experience with my second child).

Reeling from my discoveries (and with new appreciation for activists in oversized knits), I went back to my boss to make the pitch for working on a new campaign: getting toxic chemicals out of baby products. "Our fellow environmental organizations need our help," I explained passionately. Knowing that the children's toys and baby bottles angle might be a stretch for my tree-hugger colleagues, I framed this work as taking on a traditional environmental issue, toxic chemical pollution, through an unconventional lens: toxic chemicals are contaminating not only our natural environment but also our home environments. "Today's children, through the products they use every day, are ground zero." I braced for questions as my boss quietly reviewed the materials on the yellow flyer. Her face fell. She was pregnant at the time, and with one hand on her growing belly, she looked up at me and said, "Go for it."

I was excited to be spearheading a new issue, one that was becoming more personal to me. Parenthood wasn't part of my five-year plan, but I would babysit frequently for my sister and brother-in-law so they could have date nights and I could spend time with my niece, the first "little" in my life. I'd diligently worked to keep her safe from objects like scissors lying on countertops. I cut up her grapes to avoid choking hazards. I made sure her car seat was securely fastened when we took trips. I thought I knew what kind of danger to anticipate. But now, during her nighttime bath routine, my clothes wet from her splashing, I'd watch her mouthing bath toys. I was used to marveling at her cuteness, and suddenly all I could think about was whether or not her toys and shampoo contained phthalates.

In the last hour of her day, a warm bath should have been one of the safest places for her to be, with an adult attentively watching over her. And it should have been a moment of pure enjoyment for me. I had to help fix this problem and I knew my new job gave me the perfect opportunity to do something about it.

While bartending and babysitting took up my off-hours, during the day I was still figuring out how to be a lobbyist, a profession that doesn't have a great reputation—often for good reason—but one that is critically important considering how our government works. Lobbying is simply sharing your perspective with elected officials in order to influence how they write or vote on a bill. The halls of our government buildings are filled with lobbyists representing large industries and powerful companies, along with lobbyists representing public health, the environment, and impacted communities. My side, I'd come to discover, had some major disadvantages—most glaringly a lack of funding, which meant smaller salaries, fewer people, no entertainment budget for fancy lunches, and no money set aside for contributing to a politician's favorite cause or reelection campaign.

I'd have to rely more heavily on my communication strategy. I had one mentor—a seasoned lead lobbyist for a large nonprofit environmental organization—but other than her, I was mostly on my own. Entering the Capitol Building was like walking into your high school as the new kid, not exactly sure where the bathroom is or who you're going to sit next to at lunch. But as unsure and green as I was, I was pretty comfortable being a loner—a role that became solidified as I realized just how many of the other lobbyists would join the opposition to the bills I was working on.

To understand what strategies might work to convince lawmakers to support my cause, I sat in on legislative committee hearings, when politicians listen to people from both sides of an issue talk about why they support or oppose a bill. Participants in support of our side (banning BPA and phthalates from bottles and toys) ran the gamut from academics explaining the science to learning disability advocates and other "real people."

The first hearing I ever witnessed on the proposed BPA/phthalate ban was significant because one of the experts testifying in support of the bill was Pete Myers, a well-known endocrinologist and author who partnered with Shanna Swan, starting in the late 1990s (when she was unpacking the Danish study on sperm counts). I stepped into the basement hearing room where the bright lights spotlighted a small horseshoe table for the legislators to sit at and took a seat at the back in the dark, where audience members sat. I pulled out my pencil and notebook to jot down what I thought might be a slightly more nuanced and detailed overview of what I'd already read online. But what unfolded was unexpected.

The wiry, gray-haired Myers, wearing a full suit with a tie knot—looking every bit the part of the academic he was—didn't start his testimony by rattling off key statistics. Instead, he began his testimony with a simple story. He asked listeners to imagine that they were on a boat with a specific destination mapped out. Halfway through the journey, the course shifts off its original path by just one degree. By the time they land on shore, they've wound up in a location far away from the desired destination. That, he explained, is what low doses of endocrine-disrupting chemicals, such as phthalates and BPA, are doing in the body during critical windows of development, such as pregnancy and early childhood. It was a powerful analogy, one that never failed to elicit expressions of surprise, especially the way Myers told it, pausing before key reveals for dramatic effect.

The committee members asked follow-up questions about how someone could be impacted by the low-dose exposures to BPA from baby bottles. Myers responded calmly by walking them through the peer-reviewed science of endocrine-disrupting compounds and how it is different from what we learned in middle school science class about traditional toxicology. He explained that chemicals like phthalates and BPA behaved in ways that were unpredictable and didn't fit the traditional understanding that "a little poison is linked to a little harm, and a lot of poison is linked to a lot of harm." New science had turned the old-science concept of "the dose makes the poison" on its head.

This whole question—do small exposures matter?—was about to become the crux of nearly every conversation, lobby meeting, testimony, and future social media "debate" around which products were safe and which were not.

We were also up against some other challenges. In subsequent hearings, I heard many questions that would be repeated throughout my career, such as: Why are you trying to scare people? Not all chemicals are bad; water is a chemical after all. I would learn to respond that of course not all chemicals were harmful, but some were, and those were the chemicals we were speaking about. People also asked: The science around this is new. Don't we need more research before we act? I watched as my boss handled this question with nuance: Yes, she said, more scientific research is always needed, but scientists have come together, and after reviewing decades' worth of research (in other words, it's not all new science), they have agreed that it's time to act.

I also learned how hard it was to answer a question that was frequently asked during legislative hearings: How many documented cases are there of health impacts on humans? It was one of the chemical industry's favorite talking points because the answer was almost always "none." But there was a reason for that: no scientist would knowingly expose anyone to phthalates to see if they caused harm. Simply put, testing toxic chemicals on humans is unethical, even if it's the best way to get a clear answer to hard questions.

Instead, we presented decades of studies showing a strong association between a chemical exposure and health outcomes, aggregating a robust body of evidence across human, animal, and cell-based research that all pointed in the same direction. And sometimes we brought in real people who shared their personal stories of parenting kids whose health conditions were linked to certain chemicals.

'll never forget the day I met Clara.* A soft-spoken woman with long curly hair peppered with subtle streaks of gray, she recounted

---

* Name has been changed to protect privacy.

intimate details about her son's genital condition, which was associated with phthalate exposure during pregnancy. The first time I watched her testify, I noted how still the room was. Everyone was riveted, even slightly embarrassed, I surmised, by the intimacy of the topic and by this mom who calmly walked us through what it was like to raise and treat a son with a genital condition. She began by describing her son's hypospadias, a condition dubbed "phthalate syndrome," in which the hole for the urethra is not located at the tip of the penis but somewhere underneath the tip or along the shaft. Hypospadias can have either minor impacts, with limited interference in day-to-day activities, or significant impacts on sexual function, urination, and fertility later in life. "When my son hits puberty, I am going to have to have some hard conversations with him about why his penis is different from other boys and how it might impact his quality of life," she explained. What impressed me most about Clara's testimony, other than her willingness to share excruciatingly private details with a roomful of strangers, was how careful she was when speaking about the why of her son's condition.

She did not say, "My son's hypospadias was caused by phthalate exposure while I was pregnant." In fact, she flat-out said, "I am never going to know for sure." Even though research had found a strong link, each person's case is different, involving genetics and various environmental factors. But it was this uncertainty that had brought Clara there to testify. "If someone offered you two products that looked the same—say, two lotions or two rubber duckies— and said, 'This one contains an ingredient we know is linked to genital abnormalities and this one does not,' which one would you choose?" She paused. "And wouldn't you like to have that choice?"

The crowd was silent.

2

THE OPPOSITION

THAT HEARING WITH CLARA WAS THE LAST ONE I AT-
tended in which I was able to sit back and listen. Soon I would be
the one in the spotlight. My first year as a lobbyist was focused on
navigating how to talk to lawmakers without looking and sound-
ing like the twentysomething with adult acne that I was. When I
say "navigating," I mean that literally, as many conversations took
place in the underground tunnel system that connected the legislative offices to the state capitol (where voting took place), designed
to make managing the frigid Minnesota winters just a little bit
easier. I spent the first few weeks traipsing around in these dark,
overly heated tunnels acting like I had a destination in mind when
I was actually familiarizing myself with the layout and the art of
lobbying.

As I walked around, I observed how other lobbyists interacted
with legislators. They routinely accompanied a legislator on their
way to or from a hearing for a "walk and talk"—two-minute com-
mutes during which they'd make their case or update the lawmaker

on the latest developments of a bill being heard in committee that day. Because there are hundreds of bills in rotation, and because state lawmakers can't afford to hire staff to help them track everything, they rely on lobbyists to keep them informed. In many cases, this is like asking the fox to guard the henhouse.

I immediately noticed that the interactions between the well-heeled suits and the legislators appeared friendly and easy; I was left wishing I knew at least one person. I had earned my political science degree, but my classes hadn't covered the art of influence. And I couldn't rely on charm or humor—I wasn't funny, not intentionally anyway. So I did what I'd always done: I observed and I researched. I started my mornings in my car, with the heat on full blast, studying the annual "Who's Who" pamphlet put out by the state legislature. I parked in the free Sears parking lot, which was far enough away from the state buildings that no one would see me poring over the postage-stamp-sized photos of every senator and representative. This "Facebook" before Facebook featured basic biographical information on each lawmaker. It wasn't much to go on, and often the photos looked nothing like the lawmakers, who were decades removed from when their snapshots were taken, but at least it gave me a starting point. I'd then trudge over to the buildings to stalk my prey.

I quickly learned there were major signs you were a newbie and that I was guilty of two of them: (1) carrying my bulky winter coat in my arms through the tunnels, and (2) wearing Dansko clogs that squeaked as the snow melted off of them. Seasoned lobbyists were able to stash their coats in a friendly legislator's office when they arrived in the morning, and they wore heels. Crisp, dry heels. Further proof that I was green—and on a nonprofit salary—was my ill-fitting Marshall's suit, one of three that I rotated. The corporate lobbyists hired by the chemical industry showed up in a seemingly never-ending supply of well-tailored suits.

I watched these subtly polished men and women (nails done but not overdone) speak confidently to lawmakers, and I overheard them in the lobbyists' break room talking about fundraisers and other events they'd been invited to (invites that were rarely extended to me). Making things more challenging was my strong aversion to small talk. (Why did I become a lobbyist again?) Even when I was invited to the occasional event, I took a pass unless it was directly related to the legislation I was supporting. I also should have been hitting the weekly happy hours with other lobbyists, but I skipped them, emotionally exhausted from pretending to be a social creature all day long. Plus, I was already spending enough time in a bar, as I was still moonlighting as a waitress at the bar across the street from the state capitol to pad my under-$30,000 salary. Worried that some of the representatives would recognize me from my side gig, I'd hide in the back when a key legislator came in for fries and a beer, figuring it wouldn't build their confidence to have their waitress and their lobbyist be the same person.

As the months passed and I got more confident—approaching lawmakers gingerly and honing my elevator pitch, which I rehearsed with some of the waitstaff after telling them about my day job— I became increasingly aware of the size and reach of the Goliath I was up against. The American Chemistry Council (ACC), the primary opposition to the legislation to ban BPAs and phthalates, was not a professional group for nerdy lab scientists, as it sounded, but one of the country's most powerful lobbying organizations. There's a reason most people have never heard of the ACC—they work behind the scenes at the local, state, and federal levels, stealthily leveraging millions of dollars to advance the interests of the chemical industry and shape the key legislation that impacts nearly every moment of our day-to-day lives. (Most industry trade organizations, I learned, did not exist simply to educate their members but rather to influence public policy.) The ACC had a long track record of defeating any legislation designed to restrict or ban chemicals in consumer products, even when doing so had them defending the use of lead in children's toys or dismissing concerns about formaldehyde, a known (and still legal) human carcinogen that off-gasses from furniture. Their pockets were deep, as they collected "dues" from their member companies, the likes of Dow, DuPont, Exxon, Chevron, and 3M.

I discovered just how deep from a site called Open Secrets, a nonpartisan organization that tracks campaign contributions and federal lobbying data. As I ate my $3 vending machine lunch and assessed the mountain charts of the ACC's spending climb, I felt a pit in my stomach. The trade group, along with Minnesota's powerful hometown companies, had already spent tens of thousands of dollars in the state that year. The federal numbers were staggering—in the multimillions of dollars. (In 2024, the total lobbying spend by the chemical industry was over $57 million, with nearly $16 million coming directly from the ACC.)

The site also tracks the revolving door of government workers who become lobbyists, and I was not surprised to see that over half of the ACC's lobbyists used to work in the federal government. (The deputy head of chemical safety, for example, appointed by President Donald Trump in his first term, worked for the ACC for over ten years. And the current senior advisor to the EPA's office of chemical safety, also appointed by President Trump, is ACC veteran toxicologist Nancy Beck. No bias there . . .) The ACC, unsurprisingly, also spends millions on the campaigns of political action committees (PACs) for both parties to get pro-industry lawmakers elected. The lobbying group is a closed circuit of money and politi-cal power. Strategically, the ACC had recently hired a middle-of-the-road, mild-mannered Democrat to head up the organization, a man with the wholesome-sounding name Cal Dooley, a farm-boy turned congressman. You couldn't script a better front man.

Perhaps most cunning was that the ACC, despite being head-quartered in Washington, DC, hired local law firms that had been representing small business interests in Minnesota for decades. As a result, the people the ACC hired to stop these bills in their tracks were often the same trusted colleagues that lawmakers had been working with for years and had personal relationships with. Brenda, a local lobbyist hired by Dow, could easily be the same person who was representing a legislator's brother's carpentry business. Or Kenneth, hired by 3M to stop a ban of chemicals in toys, may have worked with a representative to help advance a bill ten years prior. The layers of infiltration—financial, social, geographical—went deep.

If there was any chance of passing these bills, I needed to find the gaps in that closed circuit of influence and I had to be savvy. Thankfully, my boss at the time took time to mentor me. Carol* was a sweet retired nurse who was leading the consumer safety coalition that helped craft the legislation to ban BPA and phthal-ates from baby bottles and children's toys. She gave me a rough blueprint for how to prioritize which legislators I met with and how to leverage the parents, health care professionals, and disabil-ity groups we had pulled together. At the kickoff of the legislative session, following her lead, I set up a meeting with key lawmakers to introduce our priorities for the session, covering as much ground as possible in the fifteen minutes allotted to me—thirty if I was lucky.

---

* Name has been changed to protect privacy.

Having this meeting over and over with hundreds of lawmakers was tedious, but the repetition taught me to fine-tune my pitches—adding or pulling back on details to impart the right amount of info. I also got pretty good at adjusting my delivery to match each lawmaker's vibe. Some were chatty and responded well to a little warm-up before we got down to business; others preferred less glad-handing, so I'd cut straight to the chase. Unbeknownst to me, these formal sit-down meetings would be the longest amount of time I'd have with most legislators all session. The rest would be distilled into five-minute sprints between floor sessions and committee hearings as I tried to stay ahead of the chemical industry's latest spin.

I soon found I had to deviate from my opening pitch, due to the ever-changing arguments the ACC would bring into the hearing rooms or make to lawmakers during pull-asides. It was a constant game of Whac-a-Mole. Thankfully, my tunnel talks with lawmakers were becoming less awkward. I was also getting better at being succinct in relaying complicated scientific information in a memorable way, mostly through metaphors, using the boat or lock-and-key analogy for how hormone disruption works, or to convey the power of hormonal birth control to work at low doses. (And I was traveling lighter, having found an office to ditch my winter coat in.)

Lobbying, I discovered, is just as much about gathering intel on what your opposition is saying as it is about making your own case. "Ms. Dahl, I've got a canning company weighing in on this bill. They think if we ban BPA in baby bottles, you'll come for their canned goods next. You know, it's a slippery slope," a legislator shared as we steered ourselves through the marble halls.

"Oh, is that what they're saying now?" I'd often answer with an air of knowing, a response meant to indicate my awareness of the industry's spin and grasping at straws. In this case, I knew what they were doing: BPA was also used in can linings, and they were forecasting doom and gloom for an entire segment of canned foods, one of Minnesota's strongest industries. I did my best to neutralize the fearmongering with facts. "It's a simple, narrowly crafted bill that is all about removing BPA, a known hormone-disrupting chemical, from baby bottles. We're focused on protecting the most vulnerable. Certainly banning a toxic chemical from baby bottles is something we can all agree on?" When necessary, I would lean into my freshman status and become self-deprecating. "You know, I'm not experienced enough to take on the Minnesota canning industry." I had to decide which narratives to play off dismissively and not give much airtime to, and which required a more thoughtful approach.

The hardest industry argument to deflect—muddying the science—was also the most effective. This tactic required that I get into the nitty-gritty of the research to clear things up, but the complexity of anogenital distance wasn't something that many legislators wanted to dive into on a Tuesday morning. Just as challenging was countering the "research" funded by the ACC: its own studies predesigned to align with their preferred outcome—safety as an endpoint.

The more time I spent engaging with lawmakers—and, by proxy, sparring with the ACC—the more I recognized that I was chasing the chemical industry's narrative. I was mostly snuffing out the misinformation fires the ACC was starting. While this work was necessary, it wasn't moving the needle. I knew I needed to do more. Carol had been schooling me on the importance of grassroots organizing. Like many people, I didn't really understand how boots-on-the-ground efforts fit into the bigger picture of exerting influence on consumer safety policy. Frankly, it seemed like a lot of work for little payoff—going into people's living rooms or cramped office spaces at community centers to break it all down for small groups (three was considered a "good showing"); emailing listserv after listserv of nonprofit databases, asking members to please please please call and email their representatives or attend a last-minute hearing to go on record as supporting the bill. The small stuff, the soft stuff.

Turns out, grassroots work wasn't small or soft. One informed person talking face-to-face to another about the real-world health impacts of the products they use is potent. It's not just a nameless organization reaching out, but me, Lindsay, in the flesh. Listeners were engaged and thirsty for tangible information, like how to tell which baby bottles were safer (the more clear and hard the plastic, the more likely it contained BPA), or how to find toys that were nontoxic. We even made it fun by concocting affordable homemade cleaners to hand out as a party favor. By the time I made it to the "ask"—to call their elected officials in support of a ban so they didn't have to worry about all of this—people were ready to pick up the phone, even if they had never done so before. I also discovered that nothing gets the attention of a local or state representative more than a few phone calls or emails from her district constituents. Because I had no assistant or staff, I relied heavily on Sweater Woman—we were chummy by now—to reach out to the just-right constituents in the just-right district before important hearings. Phone calls really could tip the balance. More than once, a legislator entering the hearing room before a vote would pass by me and say, "My phone's been ringing a lot this morning. Clearly lots of constituents care about this. You've got my vote."

Carol had also advised me to use the power of the media to get the message across, since it allowed us to pull the conversation out of the halls of the legislature and put it before the public, speaking directly to thousands of parents whose kids were using bottles and plastic toys. Those parents were also constituents and voters, and they were easily mobilized to make calls to their legislators in support of our bills.

In June 2007, I had the perfect opportunity to capitalize on a children's safety issue that was already making huge news: the Consumer Product Safety Commission (CPSC), the government entity established to keep our products safe, issued a recall of 1.5 million Thomas the Tank Engine toys due to high amounts of lead in the paint of the trains, buildings, and railways. It was big news and it was bad. The beloved blue engine and his friends, sold by Mattel and manufactured in China, were carrying a powerful heavy metal known to cause irreversible brain damage in kids: lead. The United States had banned lead-based household paint in 1978, but the "limit" was unacceptably high—600 parts per million—and there were no established limits for children's products. Also, with no labeling requirement, there was no easy way to determine which toys harbored heavy metals (or any toxic ingredients for that matter). The Thomas the Tank Engine recall was indicative of a larger problem: taking a shopping trip to Walmart was like rolling the dice on your child's health.

It was time for a big show-and-tell. I called up one of the scientists I'd been learning from and asked if I could borrow his XRF analyzer, a new piece of equipment that could penetrate a product to identify its chemical components. It looked like a bulky laser gun from the set of a 1980s sci-fi movie, but perhaps most important to me, a nonscientist, after some training it was pretty easy to use. All I had to do was place the gun on a Thomas train—or a plastic animal figure, or a teether—and hold the button to reveal a lead reading on the display. I strongly suspected that this tool would prove the point I was trying to make: some children's toys contained harmful chemicals and some did not, and the problem was that we didn't know which was which or what was what.

One of the parents who'd been volunteering with our coalition offered up her basement playroom, where her three- and five-year-old children spent their time between snacks and naps. I cold-called all the television stations in my Rolodex (Gen-Zers: google it for fun) and teased the event, building it up as a big reveal, though frankly I wasn't sure what would transpire.

On the day of the event, I walked down into the basement and saw it wasn't going to be great for the cameras. The space was small and dark, with dug-out windows and overhead lighting reminiscent of a cave. I reminded myself that the setting was secondary and the real star of the show would be the toys. I set up for the segment, grabbing some toys that I knew from my research were likely to contain not only lead but also other toxic chemicals that I could connect to the legislation I was lobbying for: a big vinyl rubber snake (which I suspected might have lead and phthalates), a toy tent (known for being treated with flame retardants, some of which are carcinogenic or endocrine disruptors), and other soft plastic toy figurines that were strong suspects for containing lead and phthalates. I also pulled some unpainted wooden pull toys. My hope was that they would have no detectable levels of toxic chemicals, showing that parents could trust the small market of all-natural wood products. Because these au naturel toys were often hard to find and expensive (many were imported from Europe or made locally by artisans), I hoped that toy company execs and shop owners watching the segment would take note.

Two news teams arrived. Phew—there'd be at least two opportunities to get on the local news, which everyone in town watched. (This was before Twitter—or X or whatever it's called—really took off, when most folks were still getting their daily news from their

TVs and radios.) As I fixed my gaze on the camera, waiting for the "action" signal, my sweaty hand gripping the "laser gun," I wished I'd done a dry run. What if no toys showed a reading?

That didn't end up being a problem. About half of the toys I'd lined up had lead in them, with the vinyl snake having the highest level. The mom was crushed— shared with me on camera that the snake was her boys' favorite toy. Channeling my inner aunt, I felt a pang for her and her kids, who'd soon learn that Snakey was going away. I explained to her and the viewers that there were no established federal limits for lead or any of these chemicals and also that elected state officials were working to ban two of the worst: BPA and phthalates. And just like that, the micro-grassroots convo our coalition was having with small gatherings of parents was broadcast across the entire state of Minnesota.

The press ran the TV segments and digital stories the next day. The message was delivered that the danger wasn't found just in Thomas the Tank Engine toys and it wasn't just lead. We had a much bigger problem on our hands, but the legislation pending in the Minnesota legislature would make toys and baby bottles safer.

I had to take advantage of every win, so I got crafty and printed copies of the press stories to hand out to legislators as they entered the Capitol the following morning. "I'm sure you heard about this toy safety issue last night on KSTC. Your support of our bill would help ensure this never happens again."

The success of the Thomas the Tank Engine event convinced me that harnessing the media would be instrumental to winning against Goliath. The wheels of justice were moving too slowly to rely just on my lobbying efforts. Our safety bills weren't getting priority on the hearing schedules, which were typically filled with issues that had a lot of political power behind them—legislation backed by teachers, agriculture laborers, and factory workers and their unions.

(Minnesota was the birthplace of the pro-union Farmer-Labor Party after all.) I also figured that another nationwide recall wasn't likely to happen again anytime soon—at least I hoped it wouldn't—so I would have to come up with a way to keep the media spotlight on our bill.

In my weekly chats with other consumer safety activists across the country, someone referenced Betty. She was not a person, but a fourteen-foot, nontoxic, bright yellow inflatable rubber duck used by organizers fighting to improve the safety of vinyl. This "poison plastic" was commonly contaminated with lead and phthalates; vinyl also spewed the carcinogen dioxin into the air when it was incinerated as waste. I strongly suspected that a giant duck could break through my lobby meetings. I got Carol's blessing to pay a hefty shipping fee to transport Betty from Virginia to our office. (Our nonprofit was so underfunded that even the most basic of expenses had to be carefully tracked.) The plan was to pull together my first public press event; staged in front of the state capitol, it would feature Betty, the sponsors of the bill, and a local pediatrician to speak about the real-world dangers to kids from toxic chemical exposures.

In the days leading up to "Operation Betty," I called all the media outlets and crossed my fingers that on a cold spring morning their reporters would show. I'd also managed to get a few parents to commit to showing up with their little ones in strollers—not an easy feat considering the early-morning call time and the logistical challenges of pushing a stroller over half-melted snow to the middle of the capitol lawn. But this event carried higher stakes than the basement stunt, which no one would have known about had the press been MIA. Here I was on full display in my first very public flex to show (I hoped) that I could build political pressure. Having the very people in the firing line—kids and babies—there, along with the bill sponsors would help drive the point home.

At 7 a.m. on game day, I rolled up with Betty and got to work unpacking her, pumping her full of crisp Minnesota air, and scouring the premises for an outdoor outlet. As the first legislators rolled in for the day, I tried to look as professional and serious as I could, given the fact that I was inflating a fourteen-foot duck. I was trying my best to hide the fear that no one would show up, leaving me and Betty standing solo.

Luckily, the indignity of wrestling with a colossal canvas bird would be worth it.

The first reporter showed up.

Then a few more news vans rolled up and the cosponsors of the bill and other guest speakers arrived. The legislators who sponsored the bills spoke first. They laid out how widespread the problem was and reminded the audience that the most vulnerable in our state—our children—were relying on them to do what Minnesota had always done: protect its people even if the federal government wouldn't.

Then the pediatrician described what the science revealed about the health impacts of the toxic chemicals during developmental windows of vulnerability. Our message was clear: toxic chemicals were hiding in toys and baby bottles and these Minnesota legislators were trying to do something about it. We wanted everyone listening, especially Minnesota parents, to call their elected officials in support of their bills.

Despite the sparse crowd, the press conference was a success. We ended up on the nightly news on three different channels and local radio and were written up in one print story. I cringed when I saw myself on TV. I was clearly nervous, and the camera had zoomed in on my adult acne. But in the world of nonprofit organizing, getting on the news was a home run. Consumer safety lobbyists from other states working on similar bills reached out with kudos. Momentum was building not just in Minnesota but across the country.

Feeling the pressure from the media build, I was becoming less of a nobody and more of a mosquito in the ACC's ear. I'd alerted the very people they were counting on to stay uninformed—Minnesota's parents—and spelled out the cruelty of what the chemical industry was asking of them: to take a blind gamble with their children's health and future. Now the ACC was chasing my narrative. When reporters reached out to the industry group for comment—as they had to do in order to tell a balanced story—the ACC claimed that no other country had banned BPA (though they failed to mention that Europe had banned some phthalates). They also leaned heavily on their own research, which showed that BPA was safe in large doses. As we knew, the science wasn't nearly that simple. What they conveniently glossed over was the fact that—after years of research by a multitude of institutions and specialties—scientific consensus had already been reached that it was the small doses we had to be most worried about.

After months of press events, grassroots meetups, and countless conversations with lawmakers from both parties, the BPA and phthalate bills slowly started to pass through the dozens of House and Senate committees on the way to becoming law. *Schoolhouse Rock*'s "I'm Just a Bill" did an amazing job of distilling a years-long process into a memorable three-minute jingle, but the reality was closer to an opera with hundreds of acts. Our founding fathers made it purposefully difficult for legislation to become law so that the majority can't rule on a whim. We need the checks and balances of committee hearings, where each side gets to make their case through testimony and be grilled by representatives. But the authors of our democracy could not have predicted the power of special interest groups, which ensure that those committees are stacked with bought-and-paid-for politicians (mostly via donations to their campaigns).

It was also a common strategy of the opposition to get a member from any one of the dozens of committees to simply call a bill for a hearing. This extremely effective tactic had me scrambling, over and over and over, for people to speak in support of the legislation. I could reach out to an overworked academic to explain the science only so many times. And some scientists were wary of testifying repeatedly because of the professional consequences. Once researchers tied themselves to the legislative battle in a public forum, they could come to be known as "activists," a label designed to diminish perceptions of their objectivity and credibility, the most valuable currency for scientific researchers. Some even became targets of the chemical industry. From aggressive attempts to discredit them during legislative hearings to more subversive threats, the chemical industry can make life difficult for academics who lend their credible science and voices to the cause. Some scientists have recounted stories of their garbage containers being sifted through for clues on their latest research or testimony. Others have had to move to gated communities as their homes and lives were threatened.

My other main go-to for testimony—moms and dads who were simply outraged—presented a more logistical challenge. When committee hearings were canceled and rescheduled at the last minute, a nap, a feeding, or a lack of childcare made it impossible for moms (and the occasional dad), with their busy lives, to show up. I was sympathetic, but I didn't truly understand the sacrifices these parents were making until I had my own children. (The stress of convincing my preschooler to stop watching *Bluey* and get into the car seat for a planned outing is stressful enough, let alone an impromptu early morning trip to the state capitol, where she will be told to sit in a stroller and use her inside voice for two hours.)

Often, then, it was left to me to testify. Although being in the spotlight made me queasy, I rallied, translating what the research meant for Minnesota families. My inaugural testimony to ban BPA from baby bottles and phthalates from children's toys felt like jumping off the high dive. This was the first time I was going toe-to-toe against the ACC's army of chemical industry lobbyists. I'd watched them testify many times, but from the safety of the gallery. I'd never been the star witness. Actually, I was the only witness on this day. I'd called on Sweater Woman to recruit a few moms to sit in the back with their little ones, knowing how important it was to show strength in numbers. They were wearing their "No Toxic Toys" pins, and occasionally I could hear a toddler screech and a parent gently shushing them. I sat shivering in an audience chair of the hearing room, silently going over my testimony. It was a chilly spring day, and our session had been relegated to the basement hearing room, where the heating was barely functioning. I was also unsure of my footing and shaking from nerves, that electric tingly feeling you get in your legs. By this point, I'd spoken in front of nightly news cameras and large(ish) groups of parents and medical professionals. Still, I was really anxious, as this time I might be interrogated and caught in a "gotcha" moment. Every hearing was the culmination of months of hard work compressed into a twenty-minute moment, but this hearing was different for two reasons: it was the last big committee hearing before the bill went to the House floor for a vote, and it was on me to deliver.

I'd spent months teeing up Democrats and Republicans alike with cold hard truths, like the fact that heating milk causes BPA to leach out, and that exposures to older plastic are worse. Every committee hearing was do or die, but today passage of the bill would kick off its journey to the Senate and then the governor's desk, where it would, hopefully, be the nation's first ban ever. If it failed to pass, the bill's prospects would be tarnished, and it would be incredibly hard to see the bans becoming the law of the land.

No pressure, right?

As I was flipping through my note cards, rehearsing my talking points to calm my nerves, the doors to the room swung open. I watched my gladiator opponents file in: polished, older-than-me lawyers and chemists for the chemical industry wearing pin-striped suits. They knew this hearing was important too. I'd never seen this particular crew, the A team sent from the mother ship in DC to testify that the evidence was inconclusive and that there wasn't enough proof to warrant a ban. Part of me felt like a child play-acting in a room full of adults. I fiddled with my turtleneck, which suddenly felt unsophisticated and hokey. I'd taken to wearing it on days when I knew I'd need cover—not only from the cold but to hide the red splotches that broke out on my neck when I got nervous.

I heard my name called. Locking eyes briefly with the bill's author, Representative Karen Clark, who was sitting directly be-hind me for moral support, I walked to the stand carrying two stacks of paper—a thick one and a slim one. Having watched so many hearings unfold, I had learned the power of telling stories and using visuals. With my hand visibly shaking, I pointed to the flimsy, barely-there pile of papers and forced my lips to move. "These are the eleven studies that the chemical industry points to claiming BPA is safe. You will hear a lot about these from the op-position today," I started in a trembling voice. Gaining confidence with the weight of my words, I continued, holding eye contact with each committee member for emphasis. "These studies were funded by the chemical industry and designed with safety as the endpoint, intentionally using high-level doses of BPA in rats, where no harmful health effects occur." I then explained, doing my best to channel Shanna Swan, that when it came to human health, it was the low doses of endocrine disruptors such as BPA and phthalates, not the high doses, that had the most power to turn our hormones on and off and cause problems. "These chemicals are acting in ways we never anticipated or intended, defying the outdated principle we all learned in science class, that the dose makes the poison."

Then I laid the hefty stack next to the small one, placing my slightly sticky hand on top of it for impact. "And these are the 150 peer-reviewed studies by environmental health researchers showing that BPA is harmful at low doses—the same doses that babies are routinely exposed to through drinking milk from their baby bottles and that interact with their fragile endocrine system." I slow-rolled my speech for a little dramatic effect. "Every. Single. Study in this pile has gone through a strict process of unbiased, peer-reviewed scrutiny rigorous enough to be published in well-respected medical journals." I didn't get too deep into the science, but let the strength of the evidence and the stark visuals tell the story.

A representative at the far end of the committee table started the interrogation. "Ms. Dahl, do you have a degree in toxicology?"

"No, I do not." I'd prepared myself for this line of questioning, but it still stung.

He continued. "Do you have a degree in chemistry?"

"No, I do not."

"Do you have any advanced degrees in any related field of science?" One committee member smirked.

"No, I don't, but I have been trained by and consulted the researchers of these studies to ensure that I am accurately stating their conclusions."

He closed with a zinger. "So am I correct in stating that you, an activist without any advanced degrees, are asking us to make a decision that could impact thousands of Minnesota families and businesses based on your interpretation of the science?"

I worded my response carefully. "I'm confident in both how I presented the state of the science and the strength of the research showing that children's products made with BPA and phthalates are placing the most vulnerable of us at risk."

I pivoted back to the real issue at hand and pulled out two baby bottles I had at the ready for exactly this moment. Clara, the year before, had so artfully asked the committee members if they could tell the difference between a rubber ducky with phthalates and one without phthalates, so I took a page from her book to show the real-world choices that parents faced. "I purchased these two bottles just a few blocks from the state capitol at Walmart. Can you tell which bottle was made with BPA and which one wasn't?"

It was a rhetorical question, of course. I waited for a beat, letting the silence speak volumes. "Most Minnesota parents can't tell either. This bottle is made with BPA and is more expensive than the other bottle, made from a safer plastic, polypropylene. If there is science that shows this bottle is linked to hormone disruption, why would we take the risk?"

I'm certain my face was burning red, but I kept my composure and hoped I'd successfully pivoted from the public shaming. I was now grateful to have worn my turtleneck, confident that the red splotches had made their way across my entire chest.

Thankfully, another committee member, who'd shared with me that he was planning on voting for the bill, asked me a softball question, one I'd scribbled down for him on a slip of paper before the hearing began. Most committees work this way, with members fed questions by lobbyists. As icky as it had seemed to me at first, I'd come to accept that this was how it was done. I was now playing the game with relish. There was no other way.

"Ms. Dahl, why should we be skeptical of science produced by the chemical industry? Aren't they experts in chemistry?"

I sat up taller and spoke clearly. "The only science we should be relying on is research that is independent, where the people asking questions around safety do not have a financial interest at stake."

He nodded. "And are there any other hallmarks of what could be considered good science?"

I knew he was kicking the door wide open for me to highlight the industry's junk science, and I sailed right through it. "Yes. Sound research is peer-reviewed, which is the gold standard for scientific research to make sure the study isn't set up in a way that impacts the outcome. It's essentially a jury of scientific peers who vet the research before it's ever published. That is how you know what is credible versus junk science."

It was the perfect note to end on.

I stepped down, relieved but anxious about the opposition's rebuttal. I watched one of the chemical industry's star witnesses, Dr. Sarah Frederick*, approach the stand. Frederick was a toxicologist who flew around the country to testify at state legislative hearings, reassuring government leaders that BPA was safe. She looked just like I imagined a toxicologist would—she was bookish and wore glasses and a conservative gray pencil skirt and flats. All that was missing was the white lab coat and a beaker. She began stating that she'd sat on two scientific panels that analyzed the research around BPA and they concluded the chemical was safe.

---

* Name has been changed to protect privacy.

One of the committee members, predictably, tossed her a question designed to contrast her credentials with mine. "Dr. Frederick, what qualifications do you have to sit on these scientific panels?"

She calmly responded, "I have a PhD in toxicology from Stanford, and a bachelor in environmental science from Harvard."

Great. I sank into the seat, feeling embarrassed by my undergraduate degree and short résumé. My anxiety building, I watched the committee to gauge their response. A few legislators raised their eyebrows, looking impressed. Frederick sounded as credible as you could hope for (or, in my case, hope against). And they might have stayed impressed had I not prepped a different committee member with a very specific set of follow-up questions. I'd watched Frederick testify about these studies in other hearings, and I'd done my research.

"Ms. Frederick," piped in the member I'd lobbied earlier. "Who were you representing while conducting this research?" Frederick, appearing unflappable, mentioned the name of an esoteric association that no one was likely to have heard of.

"And what type of an association is this? Is it a consulting firm?" the committee member probed.

"Yes," she responded.

"And is it fair to say that the consulting firm paid you for your work on this study?"

"Yes," she admitted.

"And were you and your firm funded by the BPA industry directly to participate in this study?"

She hesitated briefly, and then spoke. "Yes."

She stepped down and a member of the ACC was called up as the closer. He did what big industry groups had been doing for decades: minimize harms and use fearmongering to maintain the status quo. He maintained that the bill was doing nothing more than scaring moms unnecessarily—ironically accusing me of using fear tactics—and warned that a ban on BPA in baby bottles would clear Minnesota shelves of baby bottles entirely.

When he finished, the room fell silent and I held my breath. The passing of a bill out of committee was never a sure thing, and the energy of the room had shifted with each piece of testimony. I rarely got all the committee members to tell me beforehand how they would vote, so I could never be certain of our chances. The smallest detail in a person's testimony could send one or two members in the other direction.

The silence broke when a baby cried from the back of the room. I turned to see one of the moms we had recruited, wearing her pin and shushing her baby, slightly embarrassed. The committee chair held up his gavel and called out, "All in favor of the bill passing say 'aye.'" I held my breath and heard a healthy round of ayes. I allowed myself to get a little bit excited. But it wasn't a given yet. "Those opposed say 'nay.'" A couple of members registered their nays.

"Bill proceeds to the House floor," he announced and hit the gavel on the desk.

As if the drama of the past hour had never happened, the room shifted and a new bill and a new group of people stepped in to present testimony. I stood up, my legs shaky, and tried to keep a straight face. I was relieved and happy and exhausted all at once. Our team—the parents and a couple of nonprofit folks who'd showed up—met in the hallway, just across from the opposition, who were also huddling. I looked sincerely at the mom whose baby had reminded us why we were all there and said, "Thank you so much for coming." Representative Clark walked over and squeezed my elbow, saying, "Good work. See you on the floor." Then she briskly walked away, headed to her next committee hearing.

I usually took a few days to really absorb a win, but the energy this time was short-lived. With the passing of this bill out of this committee, we were only at the midpoint of what would become a two-year journey through more than thirty similar hearings. (Nothing is easy in politics.) I would testify dozens more times, usually facing new opposition flown in by the chemical industry. I had to think fast on the stand, as I never knew what the ACC would use from its repertoire of tactics—blurring the science, citing a one-off esoteric study showing that a toxic chemical was A-OK, or suddenly gaining support for opposing the bill from a new, politically powerful organization—a chamber of commerce, for example.

Once the bill finally passed through the last Senate committee, it was negotiated, diluted, tabled, and made its final stop on the House floor to resolve differences between the House and Senate bills. Then, in 2009, it passed overwhelmingly with bipartisan support, 179 to 13, becoming the nation's first ban on BPA. When I heard that the governor signed the bill, I allowed myself a good, long reflective moment to process what I'd accomplished. I knew there would be more bills and battles ahead, but I took a pause to feel proud. This was the highlight of my young career, so I gathered with some colleagues to celebrate—by now I'd befriended a few other lone-ranger lobbyists working on climate- or safety-related legislation—to toast the win and trash-talk the other side's pretension and dirty tactics. The Minnesota law triggered other states to act, and ultimately, in 2012, Congress passed a federal ban.

As elated as I was about the win, however, I was also really exhausted. And suspicious. I found myself fixating on the improbable scenario that the chemical industry had planted in their testimony, that a ban on BPA would create a catastrophic statewide shortage of baby bottles on shelves, specifically for low-income mothers. Intellectually, I knew it was a sleazy tactic to create fear and encourage legislators to vote against the bill, but the talking point kept me awake at night.

Looking back, I see that I was succumbing to one of the chemical industry's oldest and most successful weapons against progress: manufactured doubt.

3

THE LEGISLATURE

IN THE END, THERE WAS NO CRITICAL SHORTAGE OF baby bottles, but I would remember the fear instilled by the chemical industry's tactics for years to come. The anxiety and dread served some purpose in that it helped me understand the hard choices we were asking legislators to make and the fear they probably felt whenever they cast a vote. Like me, they were often left wondering if there was a kernel of truth to some of the scary stories the chemical industry shared with them. And many times that seed of doubt, that spark of fear, caught fire. My next big legislative fight— banning the use of toxic flame retardant chemicals in furniture— showed me just how effective and deceptive the industry's doubt machine could be, and the extreme and dirty tactics they'd use to keep their profit-generating chemicals in action.

They had spent decades getting their playbook down to a science (without, you know, real science). Understanding that playbook requires a trip back to the 1970s. Americans were fighting in Vietnam, Richard Nixon was in office, and houses were catching on fire at an alarming rate. Most of us probably didn't learn about that last one in history class, but around this time (and for years prior) incidents of house fires were on the rise because people were falling asleep on their couches and armchairs and beds—usually after having too much to drink—with their cigarettes still lit.

Cigarettes contain a cocktail of chemicals to keep them burning even when the smoker is not inhaling. This was a clever idea used by tobacco companies to ensure that cigarettes burned faster, which meant people bought and smoked more cigarettes, creating deeper pockets for the industry. From a public health perspective, the obvious solution to the rising incidence of house fires was to take out the chemicals that made cigarettes continuously burn. But there was a hitch: removing chemicals from cigarettes wasn't good for the tobacco or chemical industries—not for their reputations and certainly not for their bottom lines.

So the two industries got together and decided to create a new enemy: couches.

The chemical industry argued that there wouldn't be a problem if couches were just less flammable, which is like saying trees are responsible for forest fires. Still, a joint effort by these two industry giants passed a little-known piece of legislation, Technical Bulletin 117 (TB117), in 1975 in California that set the standard for how long an open flame could be held to a piece of foam furniture without catching fire: twelve seconds.. That's a long time (purposefully so) for something to not catch fire, so the bill also required that high levels of flame retardants be used in foam in order to hit that flammability standard. Getting this law on the books in California was genius. Because California has the biggest state economy, the law affected manufacturing across the entire country, becoming a de facto national standard. So the chemical industry succeeded not only in keeping chemicals in cigarettes but also in adding chemicals to couches. And because these chemicals were all so new, there was no research to indicate that this was a really bad idea. Nor were there laws requiring companies to show that a chemical was safe before it was added to a product.

It gets worse. Even though these chemicals were called "flame retardants," they only modestly delayed the moment of ignition. Couches are typically made from polyurethane foam, which is made from oil, which is basically fuel for fire. Once the open flame burned through the fabric—even if that moment was slightly delayed—nothing could stop it, not even fancy new chemicals.

Around the time couches started getting bathed in flame retardants, a promising young biophysical chemist by the name of Arlene Blum was in the early days of her career, working as a postdoctoral researcher at Stanford. She wanted to study the possible cancer-causing properties of birth control injection, but her colleague, Bruce Ames, asked her to take on a side project: looking at the cancer-causing potential of the flame retardant brominated tris, which had just been added to a product category more intimate than couches: kids' pajamas. In 1975, the Consumer Product Safety Commission began requiring that children's sleepwear meet a flammability standard (under the assumption that these chemicals would keep kids safe from fires while they slept), which gave the chemical industry yet another target market for its newly concocted flame retardants. Nearly all of the children's sleepwear manufactured in the United States contained the stuff—so much, in fact, that 10 to 20 percent of the weight of the fabric was flame retardant.

The results of Blum's tests were terrifying: she discovered that brominated tris was one of the strongest mutagens ever tested and very likely to damage DNA in ways that elevate the risk for cancer. She and Ames immediately published a landmark article in *Science* in 1977 stating that the flame retardant found in most children's pajamas was linked to cancer and should not be used. The article alarmed health experts and the parents of America and, within three months, led to a CPSC ban on kids' PJs that contained brominated tris. (Blum would tell me that the federal action happened swiftly because the flame retardant industry was not yet actively lobbying—had corporate lobbyists jumped into action, the ban might have never happened.) In short order, the chemical industry replaced brominated tris with another flame retardant, a very similar one called chlorinated tris, which, thanks to Blum's continued research, would also be removed from kids' sleepwear. This strategy of replacing one banned toxic chemical with another equally harmful one is known as "regrettable substitutions," and is why consumer safety proponents often end up playing Whac-a-Mole for decades.

In 1980, with research funding drying up and a new anti-science administration installed, Blum left science to pursue her other passion: high mountain adventures. She had already made a name for herself as one of the most accomplished female mountain climbers, leading the first American—and first all-female—ascent of Annapurna I, the world's most dangerous and highest peak. (At the time, just eight people had reached the top, and nine had died trying.) Blum also crossed the European Alps, strapping her infant daughter on her back as she and her partner navigated the mountainous terrain from Yugoslavia to France.

In 2006, Blum decided to settle in the easily trekked foothills of Berkeley and return to science. Hoping to make inroads in the field after a twenty-six-year break, she attended a green chemistry meeting in Oakland and happened to meet the executive director of the Polyurethane Foam Association. As they chatted, she shared that she had studied flame retardants, and he suddenly became very interested. "Flame retardants are a big problem for us," he confided to her when he realized that he was talking to an expert in the field. Blum was surprised, not understanding at the time what foam and flame retardants had in common. The executive broke it down, explaining the under-the-radar California law that had passed while Blum was fighting to ban flame retardants from kids' pajamas. "Our foam has to be flame-retardant, but the chemical we've been using for years, penta-brominated diphenyl ether (PBDE), was banned a few years ago." Blum was relieved to hear that, suspecting (rightly) that it was taken off the market because it was carcinogenic. He continued. "I'm here at this meeting, though, because I'm worried about the safety of a new chemical flame retardant my industry is using as a replacement."

"What chemical is it?" she asked.

"It's called chlorinated tris."

Blum nearly fell over. Chlorinated tris, the same toxic chemical she'd worked so hard to remove from kids' sleepwear decades earlier.

While Blum had been summiting the world's highest peaks, the chemical industry—abetted by the California law they'd lobbied to pass—had been adding the known carcinogen to furniture cushions, mattresses, curtains, carpets, and more. She thought she'd left mountaineering, but it turns out she'd found her next mountain.

Back in Minnesota, I was poring over Blum's early and recent research in order to convince legislators that flame retardants were dangerous enough to ban. This fight presented several big problems. For starters, because "flame retardants" sounded good, I'd have to dispel that assumption right away. Second, flame retardants had complicated chemical names and there were many variants used in different products. Most people tuned me out when I explained that "polybrominated diphenyl ether" was hiding in our dust. I understood the reaction—it was exactly how I had responded when Sweater Woman had told me I was breathing in phthalates that clung to tiny dust particles. "Now you want me to be afraid of my dust?" I'd thought. Third, no one knew that flame retardants were in our couches and car seats and textiles. The media had done virtually zero coverage of the issue, in part because the topic was far less sexy than BPA and phthalates since kids weren't the primary target . . . or so I thought.

As I attended meetings and scientific briefings, including several where Blum herself spoke to share her findings, I learned that flame retardants can harm children's developing brains in ways that are more impactful than in adults. Because some flame retardants are neurotoxic—meaning they can damage the brain's structure and function and impair the nervous system—they are linked to behaviors such as hyperactivity and aggression, as well as deficits in IQ. Not only that, but kids' exposure is often higher than their parents', not because they hang out on the couch more, but because they spend more time on the floor, where they touch and breathe in the dust carrying these chemicals after they migrate out from the cushions to the air. (Research would later show that children had an average of four times the amount of flame retardants in their bodies as adults.) For the same reason, pets are also at higher risk. When Blum tested her own beloved and sick cat, she discovered high levels of flame retardants in the cat's blood, a scenario common in cats, who lick themselves clean.

There was one other aspect of the flame retardants in question that I had to get legislators to understand: aside from being toxic, many flame retardants are persistent. This finding was so powerful that when I learned about it I began avoiding my own couch. Being persistent means that some flame retardants stay in the environment for a long, long time. Many also are bioaccumulative: they build up in our bodies. Unlike BPA and phthalates, which leave our bodies within days through urine (so you can lower your levels pretty quickly if you avoid them), certain flame retardants can stick around in our fat. Flame retardants also biomagnify: they can concentrate at higher levels as you go up the food chain. (So larger fish have higher levels from eating smaller fish, similar to why we avoid mercury from tuna when pregnant.) In a nutshell, for the toxic flame retardants we were concerned about, many are considered PBTs because they feature three of the worst characteristics a chemical can have: they **p**ersist, they **b**ioaccumulate, and they are **t**oxic.

And they were required by law to be mixed into the foam of every cushion we plop ourselves down on to watch TV, nurse babies, and take weekend naps.

Translating all of this for legislators proved to be a lot in the single kickoff meeting I had with them at the start of the legislative session and during the few minutes I grabbed in between hearings or when they were stepping out for lunch. I often led with the one thing that got their attention right away: the Minnesota Fire Fighters Association—and related organizations at the federal level—were supporting the ban because research had shown that flame retardants were likely to increase the risk of certain cancers in firefighters. After being instantly released into the air by the heat, these chemicals find their way through all of the protective equipment and into firefighters' airways and onto their skin, clinging to clothing and gear. Behind the scenes, folks like me—and the people doing the research—had been speaking to firefighter organizations about the increased dangers their workers faced (as if putting out fires wasn't risky enough). Legislators knew that firefighter organizations were very selective in what they put their name to, and the fact that they were showing up to committee hearings and testifying on the impact of on-the-job exposure made it real in a way that nothing else could.

Over the course of six months, I told and retold the dramatic flame retardant story to as many lawmakers as I could. I handed out packets detailing the little-known origin story and the strong science about the dangers to our kids, pets, and firefighters. I attended and testified in committee hearing after committee hearing, butting up against the chemical industry's wall of experts and spin doctors. I could feel the momentum building as more and more lawmakers indicated that they were seriously considering voting for the ban and as the press began writing about the dangers. I also felt the court of public opinion shifting as I made my grassroots rounds, speaking to groups of health care workers, volunteers in church basements, concerned parents in empty school cafeterias, and members of various advocacy groups in their homes. As we got close to the big day when the House would either pass the bill or kill it, my vote count started to tally in my favor.

By "vote count" I don't mean a fancy electronic spreadsheet tracking the "ayes" and "nays" and "maybes" of lawmakers. I was tallying the count on a 8½" × 11" piece of paper on which I'd hand-drawn columns with all the legislators' last names next to a plus sign, a minus sign, or an S (to indicate "swing")—all in pencil so I could erase the shifting sentiments as the chemical industry and I battled it out. One of my mentors, a seasoned lobbyist, warned me never to put my name or the bill's name on the paper in case it somehow ended up with a lobbyist for the opposing team. The paranoia was warranted, as the industry would exploit any opportunity to glean insights on our strategy or to find out which legislators were leaning in our direction.

My mentors had also taught me to never ever ask a bill's sponsor to call for a vote until we were pretty confident of a win. Calling for a vote prematurely was almost certain death for a bill, for it was nearly impossible to get a bill back on the floor after it had failed. While I could never be totally certain where each lawmaker would land—some kept their vote a mystery until the day of—I had gotten good at reading the room. Equally important was learning to thread the needle through that narrow window of opportunity when I had the advantage, before the chemical industry had a chance to work a legislator over to their side. It was all about timing.

The morning of the flame retardant vote, I sat in the old wooden chairs lining the gallery watching the conversations unfold below on the House floor. I felt good about our chances, based on the vote count I had done, until I noticed an unusual rustling of papers. Instead of listening to the bill's lead author talk about protecting future generations, lawmakers were distracted by a paper being distributed by young interns, called "pages." Mumbles and concerned looks ensued. Legislators who were in my "aye" column of the vote count were getting up and talking to those firmly in the "nay" camp. My heart began to race.

A lead Democrat stood up and announced, "An important letter has just come in from the hospital burn unit that I think deserves our attention."

My stomach dropped. No longer naive about the industry's strategy to create last-minute doubt, I knew what was happening.

The chemical industry had devised a carefully timed letter to oppose the bill, sent from a burn unit that happened to be located in the district of this representative. He was a moderate, and when he took a side on an issue and spoke about it from the floor, many moderates from both parties followed his lead. My vote count was now a sweaty crumpled piece of paper in my hand. He read the letter out loud, which told stories of children who were allegedly burned in house fires and stated how reckless it would be to ban these chemicals. The strategy was devious and convincing— dropping a doubt-producing letter moments before the vote that would ban this chemical from our homes, using something as horrible and visceral as the mental image of children with permanent scars from burns across their body.

I had mere minutes to do damage control. I ran downstairs and scribbled some counterpoints on a few pieces of paper, along with a request to meet me outside of the chambers for a quick debrief (since no lobbyists were allowed on the House floor and texting wasn't a thing yet). I handed the messages to a page and asked him to run—I meant actually run—them to key legislators. Soon they joined me in the hallway, where I was pacing and mentally running through how to best defuse this last-minute bomb. I led with the truth, explaining that this was an eleventh-hour attempt by the chemical industry to discredit the bill. (This strategy would be replicated across the United States until it was exposed by the *Chicago Tribune* in 2012. Turns out, there were exactly zero children in burn units who'd suffered and died as a result of fires that could have been prevented by flame retardants.) I reminded the legislators that flame retardants did not slow the spread of fires in couches and that decades of good science showed that they were highly toxic to humans. They nodded, but I had no idea if these key points would be enough to overcome the image of burned and suffering children.

I sprinted up the spiral marble staircase and back to the gallery to see how things would shake out, watching my two stronghold legislators convene with other members. Less than five minutes later, and with my heart still racing, I watched with relief as the vote board lit up mostly green (indicating the bill passed), though I noted a few more red dots than I'd expected. At the end of the day, the ones who mattered had trusted me, firefighters, and science.

In the days following, I quickly got to work shoring up final votes for the Senate floor. The chemical industry was suspiciously absent from the Senate chambers, I presumed because they knew we had the votes and had given up. A few days later, we passed the ban on flame retardants out of both the House and Senate chambers with strong bipartisan support. The bill was headed to the governor's desk to become law.

Naively, I thought all the roadblocks had been cleared and our win was imminent. But with the stroke of a pen, Governor Tim Pawlenty vetoed the bill. In the veto letter released by his office, the rationale exactly mirrored—and I mean *exactly*—the industry talking points we had heard at every hearing. I now knew where the lobbyists were when I noticed they weren't in the Senate: they were in the governor's office, lobbying him to kill the bill.

I felt like the wind had been knocked out of me when I heard the news. I'd miscalculated that delivering a strong bipartisan vote from both the House and Senate, on a consumer safety issue supported by firefighters, would be enough and that I wouldn't need to lobby the governor. For as much as I was catching my stride, it was a rookie move. I had to quickly consider my next play—we had a short window in which to attempt to override the governor's veto, which many colleagues told me was nearly impossible to do.

Up until now, I'd been careful not to come off as the dramatic, overzealous activist. Because so many people viewed environmental and consumer health advocates as extremists—the college student chained to a tree trunk to save an owl or the hippie mom who made all her baby food from scratch—I swung the other direction in my affect and behaviors. Adopting that persona was my natural inclination (I'm serious and practical), but it was also calculated. I believed that my matter-of-fact demeanor was one of the reasons that moderates in both parties took me seriously. I laid out the facts and let them speak for themselves. But now, with so much on the line—and with the success of the chemical industry's dirty tactics in influencing the top lawmaker in the state—I knew I had to go big or go home.

Fueled by rage, desperation, and a "fuck it, it's on" attitude, I decided that a public teaching moment was in order. I printed out the governor's veto letter, took out my best red pen, and used arrows to write counterpoints to every inaccurate sentence. The page was riddled with nearly a dozen significant corrections, and I carefully underlined the language that was taken verbatim from chemical industry letters and testimony, all of which were in the public record for reporters to see for themselves. I made copies of the edited letter and faxed it to all of the major news outlets in the state.

Turns out, either it was a slow news day or my marked-up letter was compelling, as several news outlets covered the veto with headlines like "Pawlenty Digs Deeper into a Hole with Veto Reasoning." The press cycle was so large that the governor was forced to acknowledge the inaccuracies and issued a formal apology. While this apology didn't reverse the veto—I had to reintroduce the bill at the next session and repeat Every. Single. Step—the sting of public shaming had enough staying power that in the early summer of 2009, Pawlenty signed the bill into law. It was all worth it in the end.

Feeling exhausted but on a high from the last three years of "The West Wing (Junior Edition)," I got an email from consumer safety legend Andy Igrejas, a policy phenom, requesting a call. I had a hunch it might be the kind of call I needed privacy for, so I walked to a nearby park. Feeling the first warm breeze of summer rolling in, I dialed his number. Andy was forming a national coalition in DC—very similar to the one I was leading in Minnesota, but super-sized—to reform the Toxic Substances Control Act, the outdated federal law that was responsible for grandfathering all these toxic chemicals into our lives.

The coalition Andy was pulling together was named Safer Chemicals, Healthy Families, and while a mouthful, the word choice was deliberate: advocates weren't against all chemicals, but only the ones that were toxic. The coalition was pushing for a future when we would use safer chemicals in making the products we all loved and relied on. He needed someone like me—a legislative strategist who could also do grassroots organizing—to lobby Congress for change. There couldn't have been a better time for taking on this work: funding for environmental organizations was at an all-time high (relatively speaking, as we were all still non-profits), and the political landscape—a Democratic supermajority in Congress and an Obama White House—was stacked with the party that was more likely to champion consumer safety regulation (or so we thought). Sitting under a tree, trying to get some shade, I held my BlackBerry against my ear as Andy asked me if I would consider joining him to take on TSCA.

As much as I didn't want to give up my life in Minneapolis—my family and loved ones, the steady movement on state policy—I knew this was the work that needed to happen on a national level. We needed to fix the federal laws that were responsible for this whole mess.

So I said yes and started packing. My six-year-old niece was particularly distraught at my leaving. Sitting on the carpet at the top of her stairs, I told her about my big move and assured her I'd only have to be gone for maybe two years. My words were genuine, but they were ignorant. I had no idea how relatively easy Minnesota politics were compared to DC. And I made a mistake I now know as a parent is a cardinal sin: I made a promise to a child I couldn't keep. With equal parts optimism and sadness, I hugged my family goodbye and set off with the plan to transform monstrous federal laws.

Little did I know that my promise to be away for only two years was a failed one—I would be gone for more than a decade.

4

THE COMMUNITIES

ON A MUGGY, RAINY NIGHT IN AUGUST, I ARRIVED IN Washington, DC, with two stuffed duffle bags. The taxi deposited me at my new home: a rental shared with seven young guys who'd been rooming together since college. "Frat house" likely wasn't what my parents had envisioned when I told them I got a hot-shot job in DC. As I struggled to climb the stairs with my life's contents, I was greeted by three of the roommates on the porch. One of them held out a bong and said, "Want a rip?" I politely declined. My "room" turned out to be a small space off the living room, separated by glass doors that gave it a fishbowl vibe. For privacy, they'd hung cheap vinyl blinds that were off-gassing so badly I had to sleep with my head out the window to avoid inhaling fumes—likely a combo of phthalates and toxic VOCs (volatile organic compounds). It was a potent reminder of what I was there for: to strengthen federal chemical safety laws.

That night, with a towel over my arm, I walked down steep, old, creaky stairs to the basement, where there was a pipe sticking out of the wall—or as the guys called it, my "shower." I washed my hair carefully, keeping an eye on the two daddy longlegs spiders sharing the shower with me as I thought nervously about what the first few days on the job might entail. Andy hadn't told me much beyond describing the job in broad strokes as both lobbying and drumming up support from voters in key states.

The next morning I walked to the nearest bus stop, hoping I could navigate the public transportation system and not be late on my first day. I arrived on time at my "new" office, a musty, fourth-floor walk-up that Andy rented from an older lawyer who needed extra income. Despite being located in the trendy Dupont Circle neighborhood, it wasn't the kind of place where you wanted to host meetings with VIPs. The first week I mostly shadowed Andy as he met with high-level staff for congressional members we were pushing to take the lead on updating the Toxic Substances Control Act (TSCA, or "tosca" in verbal shorthand), the weak legislation responsible for toxic chemicals being in our products in the first place. Originally signed into law in 1976, TSCA was supposed to prevent toxic chemicals from entering the market. The problem, I learned, was that the legislation had some pretty big loopholes (ones that my skeptical mind was thinking were probably there by design).

Andy and our colleagues from leading environmental organizations, all seasoned lobbyists, made the case by walking through these flaws in detail. Andy—who was in his late thirties and whose slightly slumped posture made him seem nonthreatening even while he commanded his audience—broke down complicated policy concepts clearly and with confidence.

At my first meeting, I looked around the room and was surprised to see that no elected officials were present. The people our coalition was meeting with were high up in the pecking order but had no actual voting power. Unlike in Minnesota, where grassroots lobbyists could easily speak directly with elected officials, here we had to first pitch the support staff, who would then run our cause up the flagpole. These mostly young-ish and nerdy staff members looked like they were straight out of the show *Veep* (which, of all the political shows out there, most accurately depicts how things really work).

The gist, as Andy spelled it out at each meeting, was this: When TSCA was passed in the mid-'70s, 62,000 chemicals were registered for use in commerce. (By 2018, that number had grown to 86,000.) But the legislation had grandfathered in all 62,000 chemicals—including formaldehyde, PFAS (per- and polyfluoro-alkyl substances), phthalates, flame retardants, and many others—giving them a pass from any further scrutiny. Although any new chemicals added to the market would be assessed for human health and environmental safety, the threshold for deeming something "toxic" was high; the legislation also required that the EPA prove that banning the chemical wouldn't have major impacts on inno-vation or the economy, a standard that nearly no chemical could meet. Andy translated what this meant in his signature calm, smooth voice. "Even when a new chemical is shown to be toxic, the company can keep using it under this law if it is too expensive to replace."

He always offered an example that never failed to elicit pursed lips or raised eyebrows, the strongest reaction any Hill staffer would allow themselves in an effort to play it cool. "Take, for example, as-bestos," Andy began. "In 1989, the EPA banned the toxic mineral because it is directly linked to the cancer mesothelioma. But the federal courts threw out the ban, stating the EPA wasn't meeting the criteria outlined in TSCA, which said the agency had to dem-onstrate through extensive analyses that banning a substance was the least expensive approach to protect public health." The ruling basically said that profits were more of a priority than the tens of thousands of lives lost: according to data from the Centers for Disease Control and Prevention (CDC), over 45,000 people died in the United States from mesothelioma from 1999 to 2015.

The asbestos example never failed to stun me; as I'd learned in my effort to have BPA and flame retardants banned in Minnesota, identifying a direct link between a substance and a health outcome like cancer was rarely successful. With asbestos, we had an actual smoking gun, and even that wasn't enough to have it banned. I asked myself: If the Environmental Protection Agency—the agency established to keep our environment clean and healthy—couldn't ban asbestos, which had a proven link to death, what *could* it ban?

It dawned on me that although I had become an expert on toxic chemicals in the small world of Minnesota politics, I knew very little about the root of the problem.

Upon hearing the TSCA tale, congressional staff would invariably throw out jargony Hill terms—a favorite pastime—asking questions like: "How do you think we should handle state preemption?" and "How important is it that the safety standard 'reasonable certainty of no harm' is included?" Huh? Being the youngest and newest addition to our lobby team, I was sitting in the chair farthest from the action. I tried to catch as much as I could, scribbling down phrases and acronyms so I could later ask Andy WTF they were all talking about. Often the only woman in the room, I kept up this practice for several months as I got schooled in the federal policy world on an accelerated timeline.

I spent my weekends walking around the city, visiting the free museums, taking in the memorials, people-watching in coffee shops, and sweating out the stress from the week in hot yoga classes. Finding friends in a transient town like DC can be hard, and I remember lying in my bed on a Friday night listening out the window to people walking by and talking together on their way home from the bars. I was comfortable enough being alone and going to bed early on a Friday night, but the truth is that I was lonely. I wished I had more of a community in my new hometown. The silver lining to my quiet weekends was being well rested for a week of endless meetings.

The time between being a fly on the wall and leading meetings was short. Having faith in my abilities and desperate for help, Andy quickly sent me off on my own to fulfill my marching orders. Because he was interfacing with those closest to power, my job was to warm up the folks lower down on the food chain, the rank-and-file staff for voting members from various House committees who would be critical to vote on updates to TSCA. Unlike the legislative process in Minnesota—where committees were smaller, lawmakers were accessible, and legislation eventually wound its way through the process—here the pace was glacial. When I found out that the House Energy and Commerce Committee alone had fifty-two members, and that it would be nearly my entire focus for the next several years, I felt like the emergency brake had been pulled.

Also slowing the pace of progress: having to walk the length of nearly one hundred football fields every day in order to meet up with my low-level targets. The underground tunnels of the Minnesota legislature had nothing on the walkways of Capitol Hill. Instead of two buildings, there were six, and traversing them could take thirty minutes—and that was if I was walking quickly and reading the map posted near each elevator correctly. What was tougher than navigating the Hill, however, was breaking through the wall of young legislative aides who controlled the schedules of the staff members I was tasked with meeting.

The pencil-skirt-and-pearls brigade—thus nicknamed because they all got the same fashion memo (the guys wore pleated khaki slacks and button-down shirts)—rarely granted me an audience with their bosses or their bosses' bosses, insisting that I pitch them first. They were invariably glued to their BlackBerries (the iPhone had just barely debuted) and hardly glanced up as I explained the importance of banning cancer-causing asbestos and brain-damaging mercury. For all my efforts, I rarely got a meeting with a chief of staff, let alone the actual lawmaker.

Besides direct lobbying, my other main task—and one of the main reasons Andy had hired me—was to pull together all the fragmented nonprofit groups across the country into one big-tent coalition to build political power. To visualize our strategy, I taped up a big piece of butcher paper on the blank wall of our office and hand-drew a map of the United States. Andy and I plotted out where the key swing votes were, and I put red circles around places where we didn't have support. I stepped back and looked at the wall. There was red everywhere.

For the vote count to add up in our favor, we had a lot of work to do. We needed to convince representatives in states like Tennessee, Ohio, Louisiana, North Carolina, and Texas that Congress needed to act. I knew that tapping the local grassroots organizations already doing the work was the fastest and most effective path to this goal. They knew the issues their communities faced and would understand what moved the state's elected officials. Andy was intent on bringing these far-flung organizations into the fold of the power structure, especially since there was a long history of DC-based coalitions overlooking these small groups.

Some of these organizations were doing work in communities where thousands of families live right next to manufacturing plants and refineries. Louisiana's infamous "Cancer Alley" is one such place: this 130-mile stretch along the Mississippi River between New Orleans and Baton Rouge tells the story of the failures of TSCA. The chemical plants in Cancer Alley—representing 25 percent of the petrochemical production in the United States—are surrounded by mostly Black neighborhoods, and the pollution from those facilities is significant. The estimated five tons (ten thousand pounds) a year of hazardous air pollution pumped into the air has been directly linked by researchers to elevated cancer risk for nearby residents.

The issues are not isolated to places that have a notorious moniker. Hundreds of similar "fenceline communities" (a term to describe living directly next to manufacturing) remain hidden from the national spotlight and from most Americans' minds. When thinking of the most polluted places on Earth, we conjure up images of far-off countries—Ukraine's Chernobyl, the smoggy skies in India, and coal-fired manufacturing in China. The reality is that we have massive sources of pollution right here in our own backyard that disproportionately impact low-income households and people of color. These were the very communities that had been working on these issues for decades, were important to learn from, and bring into the fold.

So on a cool fall day in October, I found myself on a plane to Houston, Texas, to meet with the local environmental justice group Texas Environmental Justice Advocacy Services (TEJAS) for one of its "Toxic Tours." Groups like TEJAS had been long advocating for the people in overexposed communities, who were shouldering the heaviest toxic chemical burdens due to proximity to pollutants and lack of representation in shaping our federal laws. Andy wanted me to learn from TEJAS and to see, up close and personal, what it was like to live and work in the shadow of the petroleum refineries and factories of Houston—the energy capital of our country (and arguably the world)—where many of the chemicals and plastics used to make our lotions, shower curtains, and cookware were birthed.

The afternoon of my flight, I raced to Dulles Airport and boarded the plane dressed in the same clothes I'd been lobbying in that morning—a wool vest, turtleneck, dress pants, and fake oversized pearl earrings (if you can't beat 'em, join 'em). On the plane I pored over some material I'd printed out on TEJAS and the region's massive oil and gas sector. The chamber of commerce had pumped out statistics that sounded incredible from a business perspective, but from an environmental justice standpoint, the data was troubling. Lack of strict zoning laws in Texas meant that many wage workers lived extremely close to the plants that were spewing pollutants into the air and water, and the state's weak environmental laws meant those pollutants had freer rein than in many other states. Rates of asthma and air pollution were higher in these areas compared to rates among those who lived in safer zip codes. (Galveston, just east of Houston, received an "F" for ozone on the American Lung Association's annual air pollution report.) Reading about the health impacts was disheartening enough, but seeing it in person was far worse.

I emerged from the air-conditioned airport and was hit with the humid, hot air of Houston. I joined our group, which included grassroots organizers from other states, and boarded the tour bus for the hour-long ride to Galveston, Houston's smaller, coastal sister city. I was immediately embarrassed by my outfit, which not only didn't breathe but screamed "out-of-touch DC lobbyist!" Juan Parras, our guide and the founder of TEJAS, was sitting in the first row dressed in a T-shirt, jeans, and sneakers. I'd read on the plane ride that Parras was a Mexican American labor activist who'd spent years organizing factory workers to enact policy change. He began the Toxic Tours in 2006 to help people understand—and see, feel, and smell—the results of the legislation we passed . . . or failed to pass.

As we moved closer to the Gulf of Mexico, Parras described what we were looking at: the Houston Ship Channel, a fifty-two-mile waterway lined with chemical and plastic factories, an efficient delivery system for chemicals to be distributed into the homes of nearly every American and across the globe. I recalled a horrifying statistic from my research: kids living in the East Houston neighborhood of Manchester, along this very channel, had a 56 percent higher chance of developing leukemia than those living ten miles farther away.

The landscape started to shift from fields dotted with trees to what can only be described as a moonscape of endless towering factories and billowing smokestacks. This was, as Parras called it, "ground zero"—the place where many of the toxic substances that go into our products and that fuel our lives are made. Benzene (a raw material for plastics, detergents, pesticides, etc.), vinyl acetate (soft pliable plastic tubing and toys), plasticizers and plastic packaging, ethylene oxide (used as a raw material to make plastics and polyurethane foam), and other chemicals produced here contaminated the air and water. Benzene itself is a major pollutant and is linked to cancer, bone marrow damage, and immunity issues. (In 2021, benzene pollution levels at Galveston's plants were the highest in the nation, with levels that were 1,160 percent higher than the national safety level.) Oil refineries and chemical plants are often nested close to each other, as many of the chemical building blocks for body care products, plastics, and more come from petroleum and its derivatives (hence the term "petrochemical industry").

Our destination was a school parking lot, and Parras led our group to a playground in the center of it all. In the background, I saw a group of children, mostly Latino, spill out of a nearby school to play on the swings and jungle gym. A large smokestack billowed pollutants right behind them, occasionally sending off a flare of flames. Soft-spoken and with an inviting smile, Parras was clearly proud of his community and passionate about getting people to understand the risks that these overlooked families experienced every day. Many contaminants in our homes are invisible and silent, but here the enemy was palpable. Exposures were felt in real time. Literally. As I listened to Parras, I felt my lungs starting to burn and my eyes watering.

He started by pointing out the obvious—that when most of us reach for a product on a shelf, the last thing we're thinking about is how the people who made it or the people living near the manufacturing facility that produced it are affected. We might think about how a soap or lawn fertilizer will affect us and our family, but that isn't the full picture. People we don't know are affected by the things we buy. Parras waved his hands around, airplane-style, to emphasize who he meant. It certainly wasn't difficult for any of us sitting there on the dry grass, surrounded by towers belching emissions, to see the wider picture and to make the connection between our purchases and the impact on these residents.

Parras then discussed the significantly increased risks of mercury poisoning and PCB (polychlorinated biphenyl) exposure—due to air, water, and soil contamination—for the 47,000 individuals who lived nearby, many of whom worked in the factories. Even when a resident did something they enjoyed, like fishing or gardening, they were met with a polluted fish or potato. He pointed to a sign about one hundred meters away from us at the edge of a pond: the Texas Department of Health had posted a warning telling people not to eat the fish they caught because they were full of mercury. In the distance I could see a couple of people fishing; Parras saw me looking and said that, yes, they were still bringing the fish home to their families for dinner. People loved the community, he explained, and considered it home. The reality was that despite the ever-present dangers, most residents didn't have the money to make different decisions.

The fact that these factories are situated in poor and Black and Latino neighborhoods and employ many of the local residents is no accident, Parras said. Companies want to build on the cheapest land they can, and because people living in low-income neighborhoods don't have the kind of political clout that gets noticed—for the reasons you'd expect, including racism and pure economic factors—companies can have an easy and relatively cheap time setting up shop and hiring workers. That, combined with Texas's lax environmental laws and limited enforcement of those laws, leaves communities vulnerable. (A 2021 study found that the Texas Commission on Environmental Quality, or TCEQ, fined on average only 3 percent of pollution violations over a six-year period.)

Working on the floor of a chemical factory is considered by many a noble profession and stable career; for others, however, the unseen and often dangerous jobs that keep our society running are "dirty work." (As I see it, the real dirty work is being done by chemical industry executives who allow factory workers to be exposed to toxic chemicals.) Many industries—prisons, waste management, slaughterhouses, border control—have jobs that are out of the view of the public and get little scrutiny. These jobs have always been filled disproportionately by immigrant populations (including minors) and people of color. This was clearly the case in Galveston.

Parras described another source of toxicity that exposed folks in his community to unsafe chemicals at relatively high rates: the dollar store. These stores are dumping grounds for products that have been removed from the shelves at big-box stores (like Target or Walmart) because they don't meet the store's chemical ingredient policy, or because they're no longer being purchased due to consumer awareness of problems they present. Target, for example, began phasing out products containing PFCs and PFAS in 2022. At least half of products in dollar stores, on average, have been found to contain toxic chemicals. Discount stores also disparately target communities with Black and Brown residents.

I headed back to DC with a starker understanding of why our weak federal law needed updating, why we had to fight not just to keep toxic chemicals out of our products but to turn them off at the tap. While lobbyists often learned about dangerous chemicals from activists like me, Parras's neighbors often learned about them through a costly visit to the ER from an asthma attack or in a doctor's office getting a cancer diagnosis, or by reading a sign next to their local fishing hole. The trip to Texas cast new light on how critical it was to put the burden on companies to clean up their act, rather than placing the burden on consumers to shop differently.

The more I learned about the DC apparatus, the more I realized that one lesson from my Minnesota days still held true: real people telling their personal stories of harmful exposures could penetrate the gridlock. Lawmakers were more likely to meet with those who'd traveled thousands of miles, especially constituents from their district. Those stories reminded them of who they really worked for—their voters back home. It was time to bring these people and their stories directly to those in power.

In 2010, two women from Alaska—environmental scientist and activist Pamela Miller, and Indigenous Yupik activist Viola

(Vi) Waghiyi—began making the four-thousand-mile trip to DC to share directly with legislators how toxic persistent organic pollutants (POPs) (the broad term for toxic chemicals that stick around, such as flame retardants, PFOS/PFAS, certain endocrine disruptors, PCBs, DDT [dichlorodiphenyltrichloroethane], and organochlorine pesticides), were wreaking havoc on their island communities located north of the Bering Sea.

Pam was soft-spoken, with an easy smile and kind eyes behind glasses, but her inner warrior came out when she described how she'd taken on the military-industrial complex, one of the main sources of the chemicals that seeped into Alaska's waterways and soil. "My father served in the Navy but became sick after being exposed to nuclear testing in the South Pacific," Pam explained to our coalition the first time we met her and Vi.

"He died of cancer in his early forties," she told us when asked how she got into this work. Her mom was a nurse who saw the patterns of health disparities in Pam's childhood community of Dover, Ohio, home to Dover Chemical, which manufactured chlorinated paraffins and other harmful chemicals. "It's now a Superfund site. Their experiences brought me to this work. I moved to Alaska as a marine scientist and later founded the health and environmental justice group Alaska Community Action on Toxics (ACAT). That's how I met Vi."

Vi's serene appearance somehow perfectly matched her voice, which was lilting and gentle but also possessed a powerful certitude. Vi shared the painful stories of her community: decades of dropping IQ scores and rising incidences of cancer, including in her own family. She described the two main sources of her community's contamination: military pollutants left on the island from bases that opened up during the Cold War, as well as chemicals made and used in the lower forty-eight states.

"Pollutants from all over the US—things like microplastics and other persistent industrial chemicals—drift up through the water and air to our St. Lawrence Island, traditionally known as Sivuqaq. The chemicals settle in our backyard in what's called a hemispheric sink. It's the end point for global toxic chemicals with nowhere else to go." Vi, a mother to four and grandmother to thirteen, was putting a face to the final resting place for so many of the chemicals that I'd witnessed being made in Galveston. The chemicals, transported by wind and water currents and rising temperatures, end up in cooler climates and in permafrost.

Vi's beaded earrings danced lightly as she explained that the people of Sivuqaq—two sister communities that have dwindled down from 10,000 to about 1,700 people (some elders said there could have been up to 20,000)—are one of the most contaminated populations on the planet. But before going deeper into the dark aspects of her community's reality, Vi's eyes brightened and she spoke lovingly of the beauty and joy of their day-to-day life.

"Sivuqaq is beautiful. Our people can look at the cloud formations and easily predict the weather patterns. We teach our children their cultural traditions of dance and song. And we raise our children to learn traditional hunting techniques, the kind that have allowed our people to eat for generations in harmony with the earth." She wanted us to get to know her incredible community—the elders, the teachers, the children—who were carrying on a proud and vibrant way of life that had been passed down to them since well before the Industrial Revolution made its way to America.

Vi's tone became serious when she returned to the main reason she and Pam were with us. She described how environmental pollutants build up in the blubber of the marine mammals that her Yupik people eat—in whale and seal blubber and in fatty fish. I was blown away as she and Pam took turns describing the journey of these pollutants—like PFAS, PCBs, flame retardants—and the connection between the dust in my home (the danger I was so quick to dismiss in the early days) and their animal diet.

Take, for example, certain flame retardants: when we wash laundry in our homes, the persistent chemicals in the household dust clinging to our clothes, sheets, and blankets are rinsed away and spit out into our wastewater systems. These chemicals eventually make their way into the groundwater and rivers that eventually dump it all into the oceans. Smaller fish contaminated with these chemicals get eaten by larger and larger fish, until the chemicals find a home in the blubber of marine mammals swimming in the cold Bering Sea.

I could easily imagine the long journey these toxic chemicals made from the coin-operated laundry machines in my Dupont Circle apartment building to Sivuqaq. "The only way we can avoid being poisoned is to stop eating the wildlife that has sustained our people for centuries, to break our relationship with the land and waters. But even if residents wanted to cut back on foods in their native diet," Vi explained, "their grocery stores carry mostly processed foods, since fresh food cannot be flown in regularly due to the remote location and due to weather." All of this means that the Yupik people cannot shop around the problem. Nor can they garden their way out of it: their summer growing season is short, and what does grow—berries and traditional and medicinal plants— has tested positive for contaminants. Vi summed it up: "Our people still feel the benefits of our traditional subsistence foods outweigh the risks. It is our identity and way of life we've lived immemorial." Translation: what has to go are the contaminants, not the Yupik way of life.

In addition to chemicals from the lower forty-eight that pool in their waters, residents of St. Lawrence Island have local contamination issues too. When the military closed up shop in the 1970s, they didn't do the promised cleanup and left a dangerous calling card in the waters and sea life: PCBs (polychlorinated biphenyls), which are used in everything from electronics to manufacturing oils, are carcinogenic, and have been linked to impaired neurological development and endocrine disruption. Children's test scores on Vi's island have dropped over the last several decades. Miscarriage rates have risen.

Though PCBs were one of the few banned chemicals under TSCA in 1979 (yup, the EPA actually managed to ban something), they have persisted in the environment for decades since their creation in the 1920s. To put this into perspective, nearly all people born after 1979 have PCBs in their bodies. Vi's community has additional exposure from an unexpected source: melting ice. As climate change melts permafrost and ice in the Arctic, PCBs and other global pollutants that were once trapped are re-released into the water and air, like a steady IV drip, highlighting one of the many intersections between climate change and toxic chemical pollution.

Vi recalled, "I'll never forget the day I found out from the front page of the *Anchorage Daily News* that the PCB blood levels of our people are four to ten times higher than the average American." It was a shocking statistic, one that hit me every time I heard her repeat it over the years.

The hope in having Pam and Vi make trips to DC was that their firsthand reports would open congressional office doors to meetings with VIPs. Their testimony was so dramatic, their situation so extreme, and they'd traveled so far, that they were unlikely to be denied a meeting. Andy and I suspected that these two women could move the needle in a way we could not on our own. We weren't wrong. My calendar was quickly full, and not with small fry. We'd leapfrogged over the gatekeepers and interns.

The morning of our first meeting-filled day, a sunny spring day when DC's tulips and cherry blossoms were showing off, a small group of us—Pam and Vi and an advocate from the Learning Disabilities Association of America—gathered at our offices. Our team was carefully curated; the same problematic chemicals that pollute Native communities—especially PBTs—were the same chemicals most likely to harm the brain. The first few appointments went typically. Sitting down with young, male staffers, Pam and Vi made their case. The men checked their phones repeatedly, didn't take any notes, spoke very little, and had no questions. The meetings felt like an exercise in checking off boxes, a response I expected when it was just me on my own, but we needed to maximize the long trip Pam and Vi had made across four time zones.

Our last meeting with a high-level staffer for a Tennessee senator felt like a real breakthrough, though. By this point, our feet were sore from walking around on marble floors, and our throats were a little dry from talking all day. We arrived at the senator's congressional office, did the awkward shuffle of introductions and figuring out where to sit, and took in the Tennessee-inspired, orange-hued decor.

The staffer, who happened to be pregnant, gave us an uninterested handshake, forced a cold quick smile, and sat down on a chair far away from us. We sank onto a couch opposite the woman, and Vi started speaking about her community in Alaska. The staffer was frequently checking her BlackBerry, but as Vi spoke, she looked at her phone less often. Vi, deliberately and slowly, described how the chemicals that were in the very couch we were sitting on leached out of the cushions and made their way to Alaska Native women's bodies.

Then Vi shared a statistic that has been burned into my brain since I first heard it. "A study of Mohawk women in Quebec, who eat a diet similar to my community, found that their breast milk was so contaminated that some pediatricians advised them not to nurse their children." Now we had the woman's attention. Pam jumped in to explain that the breast milk that was tested was unusually contaminated with high levels of PBCs.

Unlike in our previous lobby meetings, the message hit this staffer, who was expecting her own child within months, differently. The visual of a mother unknowingly passing on some of the most toxic chemicals in existence to her baby during what should be a nurturing and safe experience changed the tone of the conversation. No longer were we speaking about abstract policy concepts that dated back to the '70s. Vi was speaking to her mother to mother.

Vi noted that the Alaska Community Action on Toxics had set out to do its own breast milk research but were blocked, despite support and interest from the community. The Alaska Institutional Review Board had prevented the research from happening because officials were worried that the results would scare moms into not breastfeeding, even though studies had shown that would not be the case. The community being hit the hardest by environmental pollutants was being barred from learning how contaminated their own bodies were. It felt insulting to think that these women couldn't handle information about what was in their breast milk or be trusted to make decisions on their own terms after learning about it. This idea that we mustn't "scare moms" was a theme that would play out for decades.*

Vi wrapped up the meeting as she always did, with a statement that brought tears to my eyes. "I know that I will not see change in my lifetime, but I have hope for my grandchildren."

As we stood up to leave, the staffer said, "I'm going to get you on the calendar of the senator." We looked at each other and smiled, eager to debrief in the hall after exiting the office. It was the first meeting I had helped secure with an actual politician.

The moment was powerful and cut through the noise and apathy. But this deep connection with one congressional aide was a drop in the bucket. The reality was that we needed thousands of drops in lots of buckets to transform the infrastructure responsible for our toxic world. The unseen apparatus keeping the status quo strong—the powerful lobbying of the ACC and the anti-regulation politicians in their pockets—needed dismantling. We also had to supersize consumer education to get constituents to care, but I was confident we could do it.

The two-year mark for staying in DC that I promised my niece was quickly approaching, and my naivety was melting away. The question before us was how to replicate the meeting with the Tennessee senator's staffer with our coalition's meager resources.

---

* As of this writing, Pam Miller and Vi Waghiyi still have not received clearance to study the breast milk of women in northwestern Alaska. A study published in 2015 examined breastfeeding women and their babies on the Faroe Islands (located southeast of Iceland) and found that levels of PFAS—another persistent class of chemicals like PCBs with problematic health effects—increased 20 to 30 percent in babies' bodies each successive month they were breastfed. Their levels of PFAS then decreased when the babies were weaned.

I also had to face the fact that many aides and members of Congress wouldn't be moved by the social justice underpinnings of the issue. They would only listen to people back in their hometowns—the people they brushed elbows with at fundraisers in Franklin, Virginia Beach, Cleveland, and Spokane. Churchgoing evangelicals. Nurses working in hospitals where their children were born. Blue-collar workers, many of whom viewed the chemical industry the way the ACC portrayed it on the Hill: as a proud employer of America's workforce. But that pro-worker image, as it turned out, was becoming tarnished due to one man's legal battle with the industry. And it would be a game-changer for taking our coalition's goals to the next level.

5

THE LAWYER

GETTING TO KNOW JUAN PARRAS AND VI WAGHIYI DEEP-
ened my understanding of how people living near factories and
hemispheric sinks were affected by toxic chemicals. But I was also
learning more about what was happening inside the four walls of
the corporations producing these chemicals—both on their factory
floors and in the corner offices of their corporate headquarters—and
it wasn't pretty. Chemicals weren't the only thing leaking out. So too
was damning information revealing that the industry knew some
of its products were harmful and showing the lengths they went to
in order to cover it up. These revelations were so shocking that they
seemed to have been dreamed up by a Hollywood screenwriter craft-
ing a legal thriller. (In fact, such a thriller would later be written.)

As Andy's right-hand woman, I started to see the larger picture.
Andy was one of the few people who negotiated directly with the
chemical industry in meetings where the opposing forces would
pressure-test each other to understand if compromise was possible
or a pipe dream.

Sitting with top dogs from the largest chemical companies, Andy looked Goliath in the eye while they casually talked about the previous night's football game. I was never in these rooms myself, but I could easily visualize the smiles and small talk happening over cups of coffee while people were suffering the effects of toxic chemicals in real time. In fact, the scientific evidence and headlines around toxic chemical exposures—like Teflon—was ramping up. The spotlight had been recently placed on DuPont for its reckless and deadly manufacturing methods and widespread leaching of PFAS—the same chemicals Vi spoke about—into towns in the lower forty-eight.

Turns out, PFAS are everywhere.

PFAS (per- and polyfluoroalkyl substances, the umbrella term for the broad class of chemicals like PFOS, PFOA, GenX, and thousands of others)—nicknamed "forever chemicals" because they stay in our bodies and the environment—are used to make hundreds of products we all use daily: nonstick pans slick, waterproof raincoats, long-lasting lipstick, and thousands of other consumer products, including dental floss, condoms, and stain-resistant couches.

Even the treatments to protect the paint on our cars use PFAS. While the industry brought coveted jobs for workers in West Virginia and Ohio, they "forgot" to tell the workers that the chemicals they were making every day were highly toxic. Nor did they warn the thousands of townspeople who were gulping down the chemicals in their tap water.

It took a wheezy farmer whose cows were dying and an unassuming but dogged lawyer, Robert Bilott, to uncover the lengths DuPont went to in order to hide just how toxic some of its chemicals were. Bilott's yearslong battle with chemical manufacturers taught me what a powerful weapon the court system can be, and it also showed me that you need lawyers and judicial systems in the game if you're going up against behemoth corporations. Bilott's legal work would eventually deliver to our coalition in DC some of the most damning information about the industry's deceit, providing fuel for nearly every lobby meeting we had.

Bilott, surprisingly, started his career working for the oil and chemical companies as a defense attorney. But that all changed in 1998 when he got a phone call from a farmer with a deep Appalachian accent, Earl Tennant, a neighbor of a friend of Bilott's grandmother in West Virginia. The man wanted Bilott to find out why his cows had been dying and told him he suspected it was because of a nearby DuPont chemical plant and landfill. Having visited the farm next to Tennant's lands as a child, Bilott was interested in learning more. The farmer also questioned whether his own worsening lung problems were connected to the chemical plant—whatever his cows were exposed to, he was exposed to it too. Bilott, skeptical by nature but not one to ignore a family request, invited the man to his office in Cincinnati to lay out the evidence. Bilott had worked alongside some of DuPont's lawyers on Superfund cleanups (he'd represented chemical companies, but never DuPont) and believed they played by the book.

The Tennants arrived in Cincinnati to show Bilott their evidence, unloading videotapes and paperwork from their car. Dressed in jeans and a flannel shirt, his hands calloused from a lifetime of farmwork, Tennant was a stark contrast to the suits of the polished corporate law firm. After looking at videos of the dead cows—flies swirling around their eyes, patches of hair missing, and blood oozing out of their eyes and noses—Bilott understood that something was very wrong. The videos also showed a wastewater pipe sending green frothy water straight to Tennant's farm. Bilott took the case on a contingency fee, agreeing to be paid only if he achieved a positive outcome in court. His favor to a family friend would eventually become the issue that defined his career and earned him the *New York Times* headline, "The Lawyer Who Became DuPont's Worst Nightmare." (Bilott's battle with the chemical giant would also be made into the movie *Dark Waters*, with Mark Ruffalo playing Bilott.)

Bilott shared with me that when he started his investigation, the case seemed straightforward. "I figured I'd be able to resolve the case quickly and on my own." Open-minded as to what the root of the problem was, he began his research by looking at whether any particular chemicals could be the reason for dead livestock. An expert on federal environmental laws, he couldn't find any chemicals that might cause the type of harm experienced by Tennant's cows, especially when looking at those regulated under the Clean Air Act, the Clean Water Act, and our old friend TSCA. Next, Bilott tried directly engaging with DuPont to learn more about its plant and waste disposal practices, given that he'd already worked with some of the company's lawyers while he was representing other clients. But his phone calls, meeting requests, and letters were met with silence.

So in 1999, Bilott filed a lawsuit against DuPont, forcing the company to respond, which it did by sharing documentation that it had already sent a team of six veterinarians (three hand-selected by DuPont and three chosen by the Environmental Protection Agency)—to assess the situation back in 1997, when Tennant had first started complaining. The vets had conducted a site visit on the farm and watched the videos of the cows showing black teeth and rotted internal organs. In the report DuPont eventually issued in early 2000, the company blamed Tennant himself for the deaths, citing poor animal husbandry practices. Neither the vets' investigation nor Bilott's research found evidence of any known chemicals that would be this toxic.

Bilott knew there had to be something everyone was missing, so he kept digging. Reviewing his stack of papers from his initial research, he found that during the summer of 2000 the company had sent a letter to the EPA referencing a chemical he had never heard of, one called PFOA (perfluorooctanoic acid). That was odd. Intent on unraveling the PFOA thread, Bilott did something that lawyers often do when they are being stonewalled in a lawsuit: he filed a motion with the court requiring that DuPont send him any files related to the chemical PFOA. Companies do not enjoy this legal maneuver, for obvious reasons, as it gives the opposing team (and possibly the media and the public) access to potentially incriminating internal documents—memos, emails, reports. So to make it extremely hard for opposing lawyers to find anything noteworthy, companies respond by burying them in an overwhelming amount of paperwork, creating a needle-in-a-haystack situation.

And that's exactly what DuPont did. On a windy day, Bilott arrived at work to find the first installment of dozens of boxes—well over 100,000 pages that would become millions—stacked high in his office.

What Dupont hadn't counted on was that Bilott secretly enjoyed following paper trails and hunting for clues. Meticulously organizing the mass of documents in chronological order, Bilott started at the beginning and read through the evidence page by page. Fueled by endless cups of bad office coffee, he sat cross-legged on his floor, late night after late night, poring over it all. "It just seemed so complicated, and there was a lot of stuff I didn't understand. I was a liberal arts undergrad who went to law school to avoid science."

He began deciphering DuPont's internal lingo, sorting out the alphabet soup of acronyms representing various chemicals and product formulas. Several chemicals kept appearing that neither he nor the chemist he consulted had ever heard of: APFO (ammonium perfluorooctanoate), C8, PFOS, the mysterious PFOA from the EPA letter, and others. (Later Bilott would find out that solving this large puzzle was made more difficult by DuPont's use of six different names for the chemical in question, all part of a larger class of fluorinated compounds called PFAS.) Given that all PFAS were grandfathered under TSCA, none of these compounds were properly studied or listed as hazardous. Translation: no one was looking for PFAS in any of its iterations.

But DuPont's own internal animal studies showed that many of the PFAS chemicals it used were highly hazardous. Proceeding through the files, Bilott created subfiles of key themes: water quality reports, papers on different analytical methods used to test chemical safety, concerning rat studies showing health effects, and discharge data from the factory's water and air outputs. Clearly, it was a much larger issue than Tennant's cows.

It got worse (or better, if you're a plaintiff's attorney going up against one of the most powerful chemical companies in history). After more late nights of sifting through the piles that now covered every surface of his office, Bilott discovered that DuPont had known since the 1950s about the risks of PFOA's toxicity. 3M, which first sold DuPont PFOA, cited the importance of treating it as a chemical hazard and properly disposing of the powder and any wastewater. DuPont had ignored 3M's advice and dumped hundreds of thousands of pounds of PFOA and its waste sludge directly into the community and other holding ponds. Equally horrific, DuPont had secretly been conducting human studies for decades on its own workers about exposure to PFOA.

Bilott was stunned. It was one thing for a company to use a chemical that hadn't been tested for safety, turning a blind eye to whether it was toxic or not (pretty awful); it was another thing altogether to use it knowing it was harmful (downright evil). Researchers hired by the chemical companies had noted the skin irritation and respiratory issues experienced by workers who were exposed daily as they directly interacted with PFOA. In fact, over the decades DuPont factory workers had developed a name for the nausea, diarrhea, and vomiting associated with working at the company: the "Teflon flu." (Later, leaked documents from DuPont also revealed that in the 1960s the company laced cigarettes with Teflon, made with PFOA, to see how it impacted humans: nearly all of them became sick with flu-like symptoms.)

If you're wondering what else the chemicals were doing to workers' bodies, well, so did DuPont. After surveying pregnant factory workers in 1981, they found that 25 percent of respondents had children with birth defects of the eyes. The company knew that the chemical didn't break down in the body, that it hung around in the blood, that it was dangerous, and that it was likely also persistent in the environment.

And then Bilott happened upon the final puzzle piece: DuPont had knowingly dumped sludge with high levels of PFAS into the landfill near Tennant's farm. The report also showed that since the 1970s DuPont had allowed PFAS from a Teflon plant to leak into the water supply of Lubeck, West Virginia, and Parkersburg and Little Hocking, Ohio, where many factory workers lived. The town of Belpre, Ohio, just across the Ohio River, was also being polluted. The chemical wasn't just poisoning one man's cows—it was poisoning 100,000 people. Bilott was floored.

As weak as TSCA was, it did have one provision that gave Bilott something to hang his lawsuit on, a regulatory hurdle that, had DuPont complied with it, could have prevented at least some of the devastating pollution: all chemical companies were required by law to notify the EPA if they had evidence that any of their chemicals posed a "substantial risk of injury to human health or the environment." DuPont did have evidence of injury . . . and failed to report it. TSCA's scout's honor policy clearly wasn't cutting it.

Many folks think of our federal agencies, such as the EPA, as overlords that enforce annoying rules designed to make it tough to do business. But the main role these agencies play is one of baseline public protection. The EPA, started under the Republican Nixon administration, is designed to shield the public and the environment from exactly this kind of corporate coverup. It's also supposed to hold polluters accountable.

But the agency can only enforce what the law asks of it. Under a feeble TSCA that gave chemicals like PFOA/PFAS a pass and that relied on the companies to police themselves, the EPA couldn't step in and take action.

With all the evidence in front of him and a broad picture of DuPont's violations—both legal and ethical—Bilott reached out to DuPont and explained that what he had found was damning. DuPont quickly settled Tennant's case in 2001, but Bilott and Tennant were aware that the problem had spread far beyond the Tennants' farm, and they were intent on doing something about it as a matter of public service. PFOA was still in the drinking water of tens of thousands of Tennant's neighbors in the surrounding community—and none had been told.

It took several more years, but Bilott made good on his promise to his clients—the tens of thousands of inhabitants of the polluted towns who'd filed a class action suit against DuPont—ultimately securing a sizable settlement for the class. In 2004, DuPont agreed to pay $70 million and finally to install new PFOA water filter treatment systems in local drinking water supplies (gee thanks?). In 2005, the company had to pay out a $16.5 million settlement to the

EPA for violations of TSCA. These were significant victories, ones that made a splash in the media and gave us activists a clear way to discredit the chemical industry and reveal them as the public enemy they were. Despite endless lawyer jokes and critiques, Bilott's case against DuPont shows exactly why the legal system is often the last and only option for people seeking justice.

Bilott was happy with his wins, but not totally satisfied, especially after he realized that PFOA and related PFAS were not just impacting people drinking from local water supplies in Ohio and West Virginia but were likely present in the drinking water and blood of millions of people all over the country, without their consent. The CDC had been testing Americans' bodies for the presence of various PFAS since 1999, and the results showed widespread exposure. Plus, none of the settlements required DuPont to admit wrongdoing or to disclose where the contamination was, nor did they stop the company from making the chemicals. PFAS still weren't designated as a toxic class of chemicals because the research showing that PFAS were linked to human health problems was sparse. (DuPont's own clandestine studies didn't qualify since they weren't public.) Sure, there were many anecdotal accounts of townspeople and workers developing cancers and immune conditions like lupus at high rates. But scientifically sound data was needed to make the leap from chemical to health harm.

So Bilott took a huge gamble: if the people involved in the class action suit agreed to use the settlement money to collect PFOA blood samples, they could create that human study of 70,000 people who'd already been exposed to the chemical, unknowingly, for years. The townspeople signed on, and twelve studies were designed—epidemiological gold—to understand what PFOA were doing to the bodies of those exposed to unsafe levels for a year or more. What the townspeople primarily wanted wasn't money, but to live without the fear that they and their kids and grandkids and pets were still being poisoned.

The wait for the study results was torturous for the clients and for Bilott, who felt the heavy responsibility of having asked them to delay any medical monitoring or financial damages. During this waiting period, people were getting sick and dying. Tragically, Tennant himself passed away from a heart attack after fighting cancer for a couple of years; his wife died two years later from cancer. Bilott's own physical and mental health started to falter, which he attributed mostly to stress. On his worst days, Bilott reminded himself that the data couldn't be rushed if it was to adhere to the highest scientific standards and deliver evidence to hold DuPont accountable.

While Bilott and his clients were biding their time, lobbyists like me were leveraging his earlier legal wins, which enabled us to make a stronger case than ever for TSCA reform in DC. When Hill staff smugly said, "It's not like companies are dumping hazardous chemicals into rivers anymore," we could reply, "Unfortunately, they are." The fact that TSCA in its present form couldn't have stopped the things DuPont had done to the residents of places like Lubeck and Little Hocking meant that the laws currently on the books weren't nearly strong enough, and that corporations could not be trusted to make their own responsible decisions about the safety and handling of their chemicals.

When I met with high-level congressional staff on the Hill, I could share the damning details revealed by the lawsuits, showing how corporations were allowed to invent new chemicals without having to prove their safety, nor did they have to keep those chemicals from harming their own workers or leaching into water supplies and soil, even though they knew these chemicals were toxic. I could prove to lawmakers that a little-known chemical had killed livestock and had silently made its way into the tap water that people drank, cooked with, and bathed in.

I could also lay out data from the CDC and the ongoing NHANES research to show that these chemicals weren't poisoning just workers in West Virginia and townspeople in Ohio but nearly every American, many of whom had detectable levels of PFAS in their blood. (A study in 2023 showed that 90 percent of pregnant women still had PFOS and PFOA in their blood, despite these chemicals being phased out in 2002 and 2015, respectively, because nearly all of these chemicals persist in our bodies and in the environment.) To drive it all home, we also had Vi at our side to offer firsthand testimony on what the persistence of these chemicals meant for Indigenous communities in the Arctic. They were suffering too, despite being far from the plants that had manufactured the stuff.

On a winter morning in 2011, I was at my desk preparing for one of my many meetings that day when Andy walked in, unusually early. He was normally slow to rise and always read the *New York Times* cover to cover before strolling into the office around 9:30. I knew something was up. He dropped the *Times* on my desk and said, "Here is your early birthday gift." He gave me an intense look and a smile and sat down to watch me take in the news: one of the most significant scientific moments in the history of environmental public health had arrived—the verdict was in.

The science panel had released the first of its "probable link" reports. They had discovered a probable link between PFAS and preeclampsia, a serious complication of pregnancy that can harm the mother and baby. By the end of 2012, the panel also had announced probable links between PFOA and kidney cancer, testicular cancer, ulcerative colitis, thyroid disease, and high cholesterol. (Later studies would also link PFAS to polycystic ovarian syndrome and a reduction in fertility.) In what was one of the most accurate and comprehensive series of epidemiological studies and analyses ever done on chemicals, the high burden of proof had been met: thousands of people who were exposed to PFAS had suffered as a result of DuPont's malfeasance. I set the newspaper down and looked up at Andy with a knowing stare and experienced a feeling I can only describe as sadness mixed with vindication. "Not a good day to work in DuPont's PR department."

The results of the science panel's various human health studies and "probable link" findings were big news in the scientific and activist communities. As horrifying as the conclusions were, they energized us in a "fuck these guys" kind of way. On a practical level, the study results gave us more ammunition and momentum for TSCA reform. They also fueled conversations I was having around the country as I drummed up grassroots support for our cause in far-flung places like Little Rock, Knoxville, Orlando, Grand Rapids, and Des Moines, where volunteer groups would gather to hear me speak at local coffee shops or at PTA meetings.

We had clocked hundreds of hours on the Hill, checking off the long list of offices on the key House and Senate committees, and I was finally moving away from the junior staff and on up the ranks. Andy and I decided it was time to ramp up the pressure. And there was one particularly powerful (and bipartisan) voting bloc that was drawn to this issue and was unapologetically vocal, a group I knew we had to get in front of the people in power.

6

THE MOMS

WATCHING DUPONT'S DECEPTION UNFOLD IN THE NA-
tional news, our team gathered to figure out how to galvanize the
people we knew were powerful enough to take things to the next
level: moms. As grassroots organizers, we'd studied the history of
what works and what doesn't when it comes to building social
movements, and that history lesson led us back, time and again,
to this powerful constituency. Pissed-off moms have led some of
the biggest public health and environmental wins—banning smoking on airplanes, putting alcohol limits on drivers—of the last
fifty years. Think Erin Brockovich and cancer clusters, Lois Gibbs
and Love Canal, Karen Silkwood and radiation exposure, Delores
Huerta and farm workers . . . the list is long.

While we didn't have deep-pocketed donors to help us with
political contributions, we could channel the "won't back down"
energy and death stares of women fighting for the next generation.
Vi was a mom. Thousands of people in Bilott's lawsuits—the plant

workers and townspeople—were moms. Many Hill staffers who connected with this issue—also moms.

So in an effort to create a national groundswell of everyday women fighting for kids (men were welcome too, of course, but they didn't show up as frequently), I found myself on a plane, again, heading to a regional airport in Iowa. Slowly, I had started visiting states and districts circled in red marker on our wall map, speaking at gatherings set up by local grassroots groups. But certain states didn't have organizations that I could tap. Iowa was one of those. Grasping at straws, I'd sifted through the email list our coalition had generated from individuals who'd signed up on our Facebook page to learn more about PFAS and ID'd twenty-three names in our target congressional district in Iowa. Bingo.

I wrote to each of these people (all women) asking if they'd be interested in attending a seminar on easy ways to avoid toxic chemicals when shopping for their family. Four confirmed their interest. I was pumped, honestly. That was a 15 percent ROI. I asked about a convenient location to meet, and one woman suggested the Panera Bread just two miles from her home. So I booked a ticket. Based on my grassroots rounds over the last few years, I understood the ripple effect of these one-off meetings, which worked like a slow-drip coffee machine that eventually brews a full pot. So I didn't shy away from traveling hundreds of miles to speak to a mere handful over a value meal.

Two weeks later, I landed in Iowa, hopped into the cheapest rental car on the Hertz menu and headed to Panera. I walked in and noticed a men's Bible study group and two older ladies. Were they my targets? Nope. The women didn't look up. I picked a table that would fit eight people (hope springs eternal) and waited, ordering the Caesar salad and soup special. After about ten minutes, a modestly dressed woman with wavy blond hair and freshly applied lipstick timidly walked into the restaurant with her young daughter in tow. Yup, a mother.

She approached my table right away—I was wearing a pin with our logo for easy identification—and introduced herself. "Hello, I'm Andrea, and this is Chloe."* She sat down and pulled a freshly sharpened pencil and a notebook from her purse. We both knew it was awkward to have a meeting this intimate with a stranger, especially since she probably had envisioned my seminar as more of a PowerPoint presentation in a hotel conference room. She sat halfway forward on her chair, as if poised to leave at any time, while her daughter quietly colored next to her. I waited a few more minutes for possible shows, making small talk with Andrea. I learned she was a career woman; formerly employed in the insurance industry, she had stepped away from work after she had children. When the Thomas the Tank Engine scandal hit the airwaves, she searched for more information and was coming up short on tangible advice for how to shop more safely for her family.

When it was clear that the rest of the table would remain empty—I'd flown several states over to meet with one person—I gave her a brief overview of how TSCA was broken, working hard to not make the history lesson boring. When describing TSCA, I'd often use the analogy of our court system: just as a person is innocent until proven guilty, so too are chemicals, but they shouldn't be. As I walked through the ginormous problems with the federal guardrails, she gently interrupted me. "I need you to know I'm not an activist."

I looked her in the eyes and smiled and said, "That's okay, you don't need to be."

The reality is that I made these trips in the hope that some small share of those who showed up would eventually become activists,

---

* Names have been changed to protect privacy.

willing to pick up the phone and call their members of Congress to ask for their support of the Safe Chemicals Act, the bill that would help fix TSCA. But at this point in my career, I was also realistic about how people transition from being interested in an issue to being passionate about it to being mobilized. It took time, and each person had to walk the road to activism at their own pace.

Handing Andrea a printed fact sheet (notably unadorned by bad clip art—we made sure our materials looked well designed and professional), I pointed out the concrete tips we'd compiled for shopping for safer products: Avoid pots and pans that were labeled "nonstick" or featured Teflon. Look for flexible, opaque plastic water bottles for kids rather than clear rigid plastic. (Stainless steel, glass, and silicone hadn't hit the shelves yet.) And though I never felt good about telling moms to clean more, I recommended to Andrea that she vacuum and dust her home frequently to remove airborne particles that toxic chemicals piggyback on. I often made a joke that partners or teen kids were responsible for this step, which always got a knowing laugh.

As I met more moms, I was becoming keenly aware of who carried the shopping and caretaking burdens in most households. I hated asking even more of these women, who were already spread so damn thin. But the very reasons they were overtaxed—their proactive role in caring for their families and their frequent interactions with the marketplace—explained why they were such powerful changemakers and why companies spent millions of advertising dollars targeting mothers and designing products just for them. The chemical industry had long been relying on moms to line its pockets.

Andrea thanked me for the information, grabbed a flyer, and asked if she could take two, adding, "I wish my sister could have joined me. I'll pass this information along to her." I remember this particular meeting so well—out of the thousands I've had—because Andrea ended up being one of my strongest volunteers over the next several years, speaking to more people than just her sister.

The groups of women I met with—anywhere from one to ten—varied demographically, politically, geographically, and economically. Their connections to the issue of toxic chemicals were also varied. One mom shared that her dad had passed away from mesothelioma, commonly caused by asbestos exposure. Another talked about her IVF journey and referenced news stories about the impact of certain chemicals on our hormone systems. Parents of children with learning disabilities wanted to advocate for the removal of toxic chemicals suspected of harming the brain. And others were simply looking for ways to remove exposures from their homes, taking a "better safe than sorry" approach.

Speaking with these women on issues that united us rather than divided us was energizing for me—and for them too. This was 2012, when the new health care system put in place by the Obama administration was a lightning rod for both parties and the public and when the early signs of polarization in the country's politics would soon be exacerbated by social media algorithms. But the base we were building was diverse and strong. Some of the moms proudly shared that they were lifelong Republicans and cited their religious faith as underpinning their desire to create a healthy environment for their children to thrive in. Seated next to these conservative moms were the crunchy, politically progressive, co-op-shopping moms, all with their kids by their side.

I also met moms who were nurses and understood that the issue extended beyond their children's toys. They wanted to learn more about new scientific research showing the presence of phthalates in medical equipment, such as IV bags. (The amounts of phthalates that leach into saline from IV bags over an eight-hour period easily exceed the safety limit set by the Food and Drug Administration.) Other meetings attracted women who were Hmong (an Indigenous group from Southeast Asia); all of them were nail technicians, and they were concerned about high miscarriage rates in their communities. (The *New York Times* would run a front-page exposé in 2015 about chemicals in nail products, including formaldehyde, that are linked to higher rates of breathing issues, miscarriage, and developmental delays in salon workers' children.)

And finally, I'd sometimes find myself speaking to urban professionals who'd heard about the topic on NPR or read about it in *The New Yorker*. Ironically, some of these women who were eager to learn more about the science of toxic chemicals were also simultaneously entering the Goop pipeline, a wellness platform and shopping site started by Gwyneth Paltrow in 2008 that has since come under scrutiny for its sometimes pseudoscientific recommendations and product offerings. I was happy to be able to dispel some of the nonsense (like the suggestion that inserting a jade egg in your vagina purportedly enhances sexual health, when in reality it can cause pelvic floor problems), but the power of the marketplace to muddy the science was dawning on me. I also found myself steering women away from the elitist, perfectionist ideal curated by influencers. The last thing I wanted was for anyone to think that living "clean" was reserved only for those who could afford it.

These trips were a bit of a shot in the dark, but over time I developed a formula. First, I busted some common myths. At this point, nearly every American wrongly assumed (as polling confirmed) that our federal agencies made sure that chemicals were safe before they ended up on the shelves. I did not enjoy being the bearer of bad news, but I explained that countries such as Japan, South Korea, and those in the European Union had enacted far more protections for their residents than our government did for us. The idea that the United States was a dumping ground for toxic products always elicited a gasp from audience members, most of whom were used to thinking of their country as an international leader when it came to public safety.

I also dispelled the myth that all chemicals were toxic and that we needed to fear everything in our homes. I'd learned that when people wake up to this issue, a small subset can become obsessed with trying to control all exposures, which is neither realistic nor healthy. I'd even offer examples of chemicals that actually helped us stay healthy, like water (everything is a chemical) and safer preservatives that keep mold and bacteria at bay in our favorite moisturizers. It wasn't just at my grassroots meetings that I was encountering this all-or-nothing mindset. I'd noticed an uptick on social media of posts labeling all chemicals as bad and anything natural as good, and I'd seen the flip side—the argument that all chemicals were fine and anyone warning that they weren't was fearmongering. These black-and-white views of our chemical world were not only inaccurate but dangerous.

Second, I gave them information on what to buy and what to avoid, knowing that for the majority of heterosexual couples, the mom was driving most of the purchasing decisions for the home. When speaking about the danger of nonstick pots and pans (coated with the Teflon that DuPont was making), I would lean into educating them about PFAS like PFOS and PFOA—and thousands of unnamed others—that were just starting to get media attention thanks to Bilott's lawsuits. Though PFAS weren't yet being called "forever chemicals," the concept of "forever" was well understood by the scientists doing the research.

I explained that these chemicals persisted in the environment long after the first exposure, and that they were everywhere—in the box housing the pizza for a child's birthday party; in the stain-resistant fabrics, like upholstery and carpets, that babies crawled on; in water-resistant materials like raincoats, microwave popcorn bags; and more. I shared that 85 percent of the US population had detectable levels of these chemicals in their bodies—even those who didn't use any of the products made directly with PFAS—because the chemicals migrated to drinking water, food, dust, and the air. Animal studies had already linked certain PFAS to an increased risk of liver and kidney cancer and to decreases in birth weight. (Published studies would later link PFAS to a multitude of human harms, such as cancer, decreased fertility, developmental delays in kids, endocrine disruption, immune disorders, non-alcoholic fatty liver disease, and more.)

Inevitably, someone would say, "I try to get my husband to pay attention, but he always says, 'What's the point? We'll all die someday,'" or, "My friend scoffed when I shared a new article, saying that her grandma smoked, drank, and used endless amounts of perfume, and she's alive and healthy at ninety-eight." When these kinds of comments were made, I'd often use a visual to describe why minimizing exposures to substances like toxic chemicals was important, one I'd heard the prominent epidemiologist and cancer expert Richard Clapp share: If a person's risk for developing cancer is a pie, each piece represents a risk, whether genes, or diet, or smoking, or inactivity. One of those pieces is environmental chemicals like the ones we are exposed to in the air and water, in our workplaces, and in the products in our homes. The goal is to remove that piece of the pie and thereby reduce our overall risk.

This analogy was also my opening to pivot to some good news: choosing safer products in our homes and for our bodies had been scientifically documented to reduce our exposures to health-harming chemicals. This was all to say, if we had the option to lower our overall risk, why wouldn't we do it?

Last but certainly not least, my big goal was to mobilize them to contact their members of Congress . . . or at least to prime them for taking that next step. "You shouldn't have to become a chemist in order to find safer products for your family. This is an unfair burden to place on your shoulders—it's not like moms need something else on their to-do list or to worry about. We need Congress to pass laws that protect us from these toxic chemicals in the first place." I then suggested that they do one or two simple things to help make that happen—placing one call to their representative or signing an online petition. I tried to impress on them how much their efforts truly mattered, that their elected officials logged these calls and emails and considered them when voting.

These trips had started out as a way to check off an important box in our coalition's game plan, but as I met more women across the country, it began to feel more personal. The scale of the community I was trying to build made it hard to remember everyone's name, of course, but I found myself wanting to grow authentic connections with these constituents who got what we were fighting for. I was also thinking more about whether becoming a parent would be part of my personal journey. Watching the way these women found time for my rinky-dink meetups as they ticked off their long to-do lists, balanced work and childcare, and managed the week's grocery list in their heads, I was impressed. And also intimidated. Was this all-encompassing world of raising humans in today's information-overloaded landscape for me? Unlike some women who knew from a young age that they wanted to be a mom, I was deep in the torturous phase of my thirties when I wondered if having kids was right for me, and I was annoyed that I didn't have a strong feeling of being in either the "want kids" or "don't want kids" camp. I felt years away from finding a partner who came close to being the right fit for the teamwork that my ideal of modern-day parenting required.

To make things more complicated by layering in what I knew—about exposures to toxic chemicals during pregnancy, about how much we couldn't control in the marketplace—parenthood just felt like a lot. If that day should arrive, though, the women I was meeting were the kind of moms I hoped to be. Someone who showed up for future generations.

One morning, worn out from a trip the previous day, I slumped into my office seat, dropped my overstuffed tote bag on my cluttered desk, and groaned. Carrie, Andy's new junior support staff (we secured new funding and were relieved to have the extra set of hands), sensed my mood. "Want some good news?" she asked.

"Yes, please," I responded.

"Did you see who retweeted us?" she said, raising her eyebrows.

"No," I said. Pulling up the website on my laptop, I wondered if it was that on-the-fence senator we'd been lobbying the week before.

"Jessica Alba retweeted your post," said Carrie.

Who? Staying up to speed on pop culture is one of the lowest things on my to-do list, so I covertly pulled up Google and typed in her name.

When a picture of a beautiful actress popped up, I at least recognized her face. I saw that she was a parent to a preschooler. Immediately I perked up. It wasn't every day that someone with millions of followers shared our coalition's cause. Reading further, I learned that she was starting to shop for products with less toxic ingredients and eating food grown without pesticides. I followed her back and sent a DM: "Thanks for sharing our post, we'd love to have you in DC to lobby if you're interested." I also scrounged around the internet to find out who her publicist was and called their office. A rude-sounding young woman with a thick Southern California accent answered the phone.

I launched right in: "My name is Lindsay Dahl, and I work for a coalition in DC working to get toxic chemicals out of consumer products. Jessica retweeted our content, and I am calling to see if she would be interested in joining us to lobby senators." There was silence on the other end, and then I could hear keyboard typing. She was looking up the tweet. She replied curtly, "Jessica shares a lot of organizations' work on Twitter, you're not the first." Unfazed, I asked if there was an email address to connect with Jessica. Reluctantly, she gave me her own address. I sent a carefully crafted email to the assistant in the hope that Jessica Alba would actually read it.

To my surprise, someone I knew, Christopher Gavigan, who was the leader of the nonprofit Healthy Child Healthy World, wrote back. He was working with Alba, and they were interested in flying to DC to support our work. I couldn't believe my luck. I told him we didn't have any money to pay her for speaking or for her time (a conversation I had to have a lot), so while we'd have loved to host her, she was going to have to make the trip out of the goodness of her heart. Understanding the nonprofit world, he replied, "It shouldn't be a problem."

A few months later, Jessica arrived in DC, eight months pregnant, in four-inch heels (I told her to wear comfortable shoes), and ready to lobby for the Safe Chemicals Act. The fact that she was pregnant—a vulnerable window when toxic chemicals can alter the course of fetal development—told me that she would be a powerful spokesperson for this issue and was likely to remain invested in this topic as her family grew. I knew Hollywood opened doors, but I had no idea how wide they'd swing open. That day (and that day alone) we met only with senators—not their senior staff. I found myself in the White House Cabinet Room, where famous pictures of every president meeting with their cabinet are taken and where Jessica shared her personal story as a mom. She spoke passionately about how the market wasn't providing nearly enough solutions for consumers who were looking for cleaner products and about the desperate need for tighter regulations to steer companies in a safe direction. She was able to show everyone we were lobbying that this issue had hit a critical pop culture tipping point.

A press conference we hosted for her visit (featuring both the prominent pediatrician Dr. Leonardo Trasande, who had been on the forefront of this issue, and the head of the American Nurses Association) generated millions of press hits in just forty-eight hours. A year later, Alba and Gavigan would go on to launch the Honest Company to address the marketplace dearth of products made without toxic chemicals, especially baby shampoo and laundry detergent and diapers that she could use with her children knowing they were safe. (The Honest Company is now listed on the Nasdaq, having gone public in 2021.) Momentum was building, and the press as well as the ACC were now on high alert.

Alba's involvement wasn't the only factor pushing our efforts forward. The response to our lobbying meetings began to shift as representatives heard from more constituents back home. Little did I know that my meetings over soup in a bread bowl would pay off this quickly. Once closed off, staffers were now asking more questions as they felt the political pressure growing from our mom network.

We noticed the change, and my guess is that the ACC's lobby team did too. As a counterpoint to our crescendo, the chemical industry went to the tried-and-true book of industry tactics and began to form what are called "front groups." Front groups—also known as "astroturf" organizations because they are fake grassroots (get it?)—purport to be independent and charitable when in reality they serve the interests of the industry that created them and are funded by the industry.

I learned about their latest mom-focused front group one afternoon from a congressional staffer I was lobbying, who asked me what I thought about the new family coalition working on this issue. Curious, I asked, "Which coalition?" We were the only game in town that I knew of.

The staffer looked at me and with a straight face said, "It's called Kids + Chemical Safety."

Already suspicious based on the name, I headed back to the office and pulled up the website. Kids + Chemical Safety had all the hallmarks of an industry-backed group. With its strategically chosen name, it ranked high in Google search results. (The ACC had also been purchasing ads against our coalition name and all relevant keywords—"safety," "kids," "family," "moms," "toxic"—stealing precious web traffic. The tactic was somewhat effective, as we clearly had no money to get into the Google ad-buying game.)

The webpage was covered in pictures of children playing and families smiling, and the logo was kid-inspired with primary colors. The group was positioned as an independent organization to "clear up the facts" about chemicals in products. The resources included a cunning mix of information: amid traditional tips for avoiding lead in old paint, eliminating choking hazards, and ensuring car seat safety was information that reassured parents that BPA was safe (it's not), that there was no science to warrant concerns about low doses of hormone disruptors (there is), and that preservatives played an important role in personal care products (we agreed—and just wanted action on the toxic ones). In tiny print I saw that the website was run by one of the oldest and most notorious front groups around, Toxicology Excellence for Risk Assessment (TERA), founded in 1995.

Over the years, TERA had worked hard to show that the

majority of its funding allegedly came from non-industry sources. But going a few clicks deeper, you'd find that the American Petroleum Institute, a huge industry player, was a corporate sponsor of not only TERA but of front groups TERA had created, such as Kids + Chemical Safety. These groups were all entangled, feeding into each other's spin and platforms. The clear danger they presented was that the average mom doing a quick Google search could easily land on one of these sites and believe the misleading information. It made me think back to something a chemical industry lobbyist said to me early in my career during a hearing: "Please stop scaring moms." How about stop lying to moms?

The only silver lining of this deceptive new front group? It showed that our movement of bipartisan moms was being seen as a powerful force and the industry was having to work harder to subvert and co-opt our growing influence. We now had, for the first time, the upper hand.

Despite the growing political force of our moms—in fact because of it—we couldn't rest. The ACC still had a deep impact on both political parties, dampening any political appetite for reform. This two-party problem was not something I'd expected when I first arrived in DC, for it's no secret that Democrats tend to be more willing to regulate polluting industries. Nearly every federal bill introduced in recent decades to rein in corporate offenders was championed by a Democrat.

It's also no secret that Republicans historically champion the interests of business no matter what, blocking regulations under the banner of "small government." What I wasn't prepared for, however, was the solidly bipartisan resistance to TSCA reform. Many Democrats I lobbied were as culpable as Republicans, just for different reasons. Dems were so scared of appearing anti-business and intent on getting corporate buy-in that they became paralyzed and were waiting for us—Andy and the coalition's core leadership team—to cut a deal with the ACC before signing on to anything. And those negotiations between David and Goliath? It wasn't going well. The talks that Andy and coalition leaders were having with the industry—including the hiring of third-party moderators who tried to find a middle ground for compromise—were stalling out.

Luckily, after a year of doing my grassroots circuit, my spreadsheet of pro-safety constituents was well populated. Leveraging a strategy used by one of the OG mom activists in our movement—Lois Gibbs, the force behind the cleanup of New York's Love Canal, a community notoriously built on top of a toxic waste dump—we started planning a mom march for change. Our march would be a stroller brigade. I knew from the success of Betty the duck that schtick works and that grabbing the media's attention would build on the momentum. We would bring in hundreds of parents from around the country, with different backgrounds and political stripes—many of them teed up from my visits to far-flung Starbucks, Caribou, and Dunkin' Donuts shops—to march for the Safe Chemicals Act in the nation's capital. This action would make it clear that it's kids who are first up in the firing line. So many of the products delivering toxic chemicals are made specifically for children (nap pads for day-care providers, car seats, astroturf on junior soccer fields), and their growing bodies bear the brunt.

I spent months lining up the event's itinerary. We asked the Democratic senators sponsoring the legislation—including the lead author, Senator Lautenberg—to speak about TSCA's weakness and the need to pass reform. (No Republicans agreed to speak at the event, and believe me, we tried.) The L Word actress Jennifer Beals agreed to come speak—she'd taken up our cause when she learned about the toxic chemicals in the crumb-rubber field her daughter played on at recess. I arranged national media reporting and local media coverage in the towns that our two hundred participants were traveling from. I'd even rented dozens of strollers so out-of-town parents wouldn't have to lug theirs around.

On a sunny, warm May morning in 2012, I carried three heavy boxes filled with signed petitions (wrapped in big red bows) down the extra-long escalator of the DuPont Circle Metro stop and shuffled my way onto the train. I knew exactly what this kind of day would entail: lots of walking, lifting, endless questions from the march participants . . . but totally worth it because a whole lot of people would leave inspired. Arriving at the Capitol Hill lawn, the anxiety started to set in. Would the stroller delivery guy arrive on time? He did, thank goodness, pulling up to the curb and dropping off dozens of strollers before peeling out to avoid getting a ticket. Capitol police are strict about strange vans making unusual pit stops.

I stared at the strollers. I pulled the handle of the first stroller and pressed some buttons, shaking it and waiting for the thing to open. Nothing happened. I tried another one. Nothing. My anxiety level shot up.

An early arrival, Leslie from Virginia Beach, rushed over and started opening the strollers with ease. She had the mom magic. "This is a lot harder when you have a baby in the other arm," she said. More people arrived and helped load strollers with stacks of signed petitions. Eager coalition partners and speakers turned up— the Hill was buzzing.

The event was a roaring success. The Panera Bread moms showed up, including timid Andrea, the only one from Iowa. She even lobbied with me later that day. Pam and Vi were there. Cancer survivors and health care practitioners joined in. CNN aired the event, and local affiliates picked it up, showing the march of moms pushing strollers toward the Capitol shouting the classic protest ditty, "Hey hey! Ho ho! Toxic chemicals have got to go!"

Following the event, we secured more meetings than we ever had before—and not just with the staff, but with the elected officials themselves. By the end of the day, we had completed over one hundred meetings. I walked back to the Metro station completely wrung out, but it was the best kind of exhaustion. On the train ride home, I looked at my phone as text messages rolled in from the moms, reflecting on the day.

"I feel like we made an impact."

"My feet hurt but wow was today worth it, can't wait to tell my kids."

And Andrea texted me, "I might be an activist after all."

I smiled and got teary-eyed as my stop came up, thinking about how these women were literally parenting all of us, in a sense. It's true that they were motivated by their own children's health and future—and there is no greater fire starter—but it's also true that they were doing the hard work that every American would benefit from. And they were the ones with the least amount of time to spare.

We'd successfully rallied the moms. Now we had to tackle the front groups, the ones spreading misinformation.

To fight poison with poison, we drew inspiration (literally) from the most notorious Big Tobacco ad campaign ever: Joe Camel, the cartoon animal used to sell cigarettes to kids. We hired an artist to sketch a camel that, instead of having a pack of cigarettes in his pocket, was holding a beaker with a bubbling green substance spilling out. We named him Joe Chemical, made flyers and put up social media posts featuring the well-dressed animal—his suit and bow tie mirrored the attire of slick chemical industry execs—and blasted the campaign to Hill staff and the press.

The message was clear: the seemingly wholesome, pro-America, and pro-jobs ACC was a wolf (er, camel) in sheep's clothing. The ACC responded by calling us "extreme" in the press, a word that the chemical industry had been using for years to paint us as fearful "chema-phobes" who were unnecessarily scaring parents and pregnant women. But ultimately, our campaign worked. Thanks to the form emails we crafted for coalition members to mail to their members of Congress about the industry's duplicitous tactics, the articles written by our nonprofit partners about the astroturf groups, and the calls made by the network of mom bloggers I pulled together to put Joe Chemical on blast, the ACC had to reverse course.

The chemical industry looked pretty bad to Hill staff who saw the press, so the front groups walked back the language on their websites and even removed some material. A front group for the flame retardant industry, Citizens for Fire Safety, had to delete the flat-out lie that it was working with the International Association of Fire Fighters (IAFF) and a federal agency on creating safer flame retardants (not true). Between our Joe Chemical campaign and the *Chicago Tribune*'s award-winning four-part exposé in 2012 outing the fire safety astroturf group and chemical industry players, both of these front groups fizzled out.

Today neither has a website or a political presence.

Meanwhile, TSCA conversations were getting increasingly tense on Capitol Hill. The friendly "we can get this done through negotiation" tone had faded. Unsure if policy negotiations with Hill staff would result in public health wins, we were forced to partner with leaders in the marketplace. And our sights were set on players who had power and scale: retailers.

The marketplace was about to drastically change, and so was my career trajectory.

7

THE CEO

IN 2014, ABOUT A YEAR AFTER THE JOE CHEMICAL launch, I was hoofing it to Shake Shack when my cell phone rang. Pausing on the hot sidewalk and stepping aside to avoid the busy foot traffic, I looked at the incoming call. It was a number I didn't recognize. Caught between badly wanting to scarf a burger and fries to remedy my stress levels (it had been one of those weeks) and thinking it could be an important call from a coalition member, I did the unthinkable: I answered the phone.

It was a former colleague who'd switched to the private sector and was wondering if I knew any talent with strong advocacy chops, someone who could build a grassroots network for a clean beauty brand.

I did know someone: me. Activism is exhausting work, and this woman was catching me on a day when I felt particularly beaten down. Burnout wasn't the only thing stoking my interest in a change to the private sector. Since landing in DC, I'd watched the market for green (aka eco-friendly) products and clean (aka nontoxic) products scale in a big way. The nontoxic household cleaner market alone brought in $600 million in revenue in the United States in 2015 and would reach $5.86 billion in 2023. Thanks to the popularity of organic food companies like Annie's Organic and Stonyfield and sustainable product companies like Patagonia and Seventh Generation, green and clean brands were no longer niche but staples in kitchens and laundry rooms across the country.

Glass alternatives to plastic food storage containers had started lining the aisles of Costco, Target, and Walmart. Reusable stainless steel water bottles were becoming trendy (but not yet a fashion accessory—no one could have predicted the Stanley tumbler craze that boosted the company's sales to nearly half a billion in 2022). And in a far cry from the early days when people's eyes glazed over when I said "bisphenol A," children's toys were being labeled "BPA free" or "phthalate free." While private businesses weren't going to entirely solve the problem, they could certainly move the needle.

Notably absent in the clean market growth, however, was the beauty aisle, which hadn't benefited nearly as much from scientists' microscopes or the press about safety issues. The industry needed a big push. For all these reasons, I was willing to entertain something I never thought I'd do: crossing over into corporate America.

Two days later I was on a Skype call with the founder and CEO of Beautycounter, Gregg Renfrew, who had formed the clean beauty company less than a year before. Mere minutes into the call I saw that she got it. "I know I can't reach every person, but whether we like it or not, people listen to brands. I want to use the power of people selling and buying our products to help pass laws that protect us from toxic chemicals in beauty products." I listened to Gregg speed-talk, rattling off (accurate) stats and the failures of the Food, Drug, and Cosmetic Act of 1938 (FDCA), which was the law that oversaw personal care and beauty product safety.

While TSCA was the primary law overseeing the safety of chemicals before they entered the market (and before being added to household products like couches, cleaners, and textiles), the FDCA was responsible for the safety of cosmetics and personal care items as finished products. To make matters more confusing, the EPA oversaw TSCA and the FDA oversaw FDCA. These various laws and government agencies monitoring it all (and I use "monitoring" very loosely) were complicated, but to my surprise, Gregg was acronym-fluent.

I realized this fiery New Yorker–turned-Angelino was exactly who the movement needed to energize a fleet of health-conscious women. (I was also grateful for the poor quality of the Skype call— she couldn't see me all that well, sitting in my too-warm office with beads of sweat forming on my upper lip.) She was outraged by the lack of federal initiative to make beauty products safer— there'd been zero progress since 1938 (not a typo). Thousands of toxic chemicals were legally allowed to be used in beauty products (like high amounts of formaldehyde used in hair relaxers), and the ingredients in product categories like fragrances and professional salon products were kept secret.

No CEO I'd ever spoken to (as I often did when building our coalition in DC) knew these facts. Gregg was speaking as if she'd gone to policy school. As a mom of three, she shared that she herself had fallen prey to "greenwashing," the term used to describe a company misleading consumers through words or branding that convey safety or sustainability without actually backing up the claims. Because none of these kinds of claims are regulated, brands can slap terms like "nature made" and "green" on their products regardless of what's actually in them. Gregg had looked up her kid's "natural" body wash in the "Skin Deep" database of the Environmental Working Group (EWG), only to see it ranked an 8.

(The website ranks ingredients and beauty products for safety: 1 is the best, 10 the worst.)

"How are consumers supposed to know what's safe when the product comes in an earth-toned bottle and uses wholesome words like 'oatmeal'?" she asked rhetorically. Greenwashing had been growing right along with the clean market. It was becoming harder and harder for people like Gregg who wanted to spend their money on items that actually lived up to their claims. Consumers essentially had to outsmart sophisticated marketing messaging dreamed up by the Madison Avenue advertising teams hired by the big consumer brands. It was a word game no one had signed up to play.

Gregg hadn't always been passionate about beauty products, but she started to notice trends within her social circle that were mirrored in national statistics: more and more of her friends struggled with infertility, and a close friend and her father passed away from cancer. She began to study the evolving science that pointed to the role of toxic chemicals in some of these conditions. "The problem was that when I started being more mindful of what I brought into my home, like switching from plastic to glass and ditching toxic cleaning products, I couldn't find safe and effective beauty products," she shared. "It doesn't matter how clean something is if it doesn't work. I want a safe lipstick, but I still want to look sexy on a date with my husband."

Gregg knew there was white space for a brand to make beauty products that worked and were packaged in a fun, non-crunchy way (no shade if that's your thing), but that used safer ingredients. The vast majority of the "clean" beauty market at the time was either conventional products marketed as "natural" without being so or a few tiny brands that were trying to be clean but that didn't work nearly as well as the industry incumbents. Having never worked in the beauty industry, Gregg was willing to shake it up and do things differently.

In 2010 she began conceptualizing Beautycounter, working with product safety experts and celebrity makeup artists to craft formulations, and in 2013 she launched the company with a small assortment of products—including a rosewater spray that she'd had to reformulate almost instantly because of mold (the preservative they'd chosen wasn't up to snuff). "We had to go back to the drawing board," she explained, "but because we'd already started selling it, I decided to share the ups and downs of what it takes to make safer products with our customers. People say they want 'preservative-free' products, but trust me, you still want a well-preserved product. . . . .What people really need is just a safer preservative."

This type of transparency and unapologetically science-first approach was an uncommon practice at the time. I loved how Gregg was doing business differently and was willing to share when the company made mistakes. That took guts and was something I was looking for (as were millions of other Americans) from the brands I purchased.

Nearly two hours into the conversation—and still grateful for the crappy Skype quality, since boob sweat was now visible on my white shirt—I finished explaining all the roles I played in our work in DC. Gregg asked, "How do you have time to do all that?"

Deadpan, I answered, "I don't have much of a social life."

Responding with a staccato laugh I would come to know well, she said, "You and me both." I had a feeling that despite being very different people (with exceedingly different wardrobes—her pressed button-down white shirt and stylish glasses were understated and classy), we would hit it off.

Wrapping up, Gregg said, "I know how to start a company, but I don't know how to navigate Washington. I need someone like you to help mobilize this army of women we are building to become advocates for change." By "army" she meant the people selling Beautycounter products, the women representing the brand with their loyal customer base. Beautycounter was sold through various channels—including traditional brick-and-mortar stores and online retail—as well as through a network of salespeople who spoke directly with customers. "I want to train them on how to do what you do, to push our lawmakers to pass cosmetic safety laws that do what they are supposed to do: actually keep us safe."

Excited about the potential of this new avenue, I sat back in my chair and felt a swirl of energy and a large pang of fear, knowing the realities associated with leaving Andy and our coalition's work. Andy had become a close friend and was increasingly facing health issues related to the stress of work and keeping everyone motivated. I worried not only about Andy losing the support of a right-hand operator like myself but also about the coalition. Once aligned around a shared vision, it was now held together, in Andy's words, "by bubble gum and paper clips." But I also knew that TSCA reform was imminent and that Gregg, who would play well with the DC crowd, could get us to that tipping point sooner rather than later. Having a polished CEO making some of the arguments versus me, a lobbyist, would lend freshness and serious credibility to the issue. Whether I liked it or not, Hill staff and members of Congress of all political stripes listened to companies and CEOs—especially CEOs of fast-growing and profitable companies. (Beautycounter was lightning out of the gate, and though it wasn't yet pulling in big numbers, it would—to the tune of $400 million in sales in 2022.) Activism itself needed a makeover, and she was the perfect face for it.

I was also envisioning the potential of educating women through a consumer brand, a reach that would extend far beyond my flights around the country to meetups in sandwich shops and church basements. That, and the idea of working on something new—cosmetics reform, which was next in line for consumer safety legislation after TSCA—excited me. So I called Gregg's assistant to set up the rounds of on-site interviews.

Landing in Los Angeles, I checked into a nice hotel, blocks away from the office, and I was already imagining what it might be like to live amid sunshine and palm trees. The next morning I walked in ready for a full day of interviews, wearing new pink high heels that were too tall and slippery on the polished concrete floor of the Santa Monica open-floor-plan office. Fresh white flowers were placed throughout the space, and free kombucha was in the fridge. As I walked past a few employees in casual but put-together outfits and designer sneakers, I realized my navy suit and pumps were not "on brand" for LA.

The interviews went well, but two things became super clear after eight hours of talking with the lean startup team: they had no idea what I actually did and how I would fit into the business; and it would be a steep learning curve for me to assimilate into corporate culture.

As I made my way through the process, I also grappled with the fear of leaving the credible mantle of an independent nonprofit and worried about the optics of "selling out" by going to corporate America. I liked being the agitator on the outside. Plus, we were having some success in molding the marketplace. We'd pushed several retailers, including Walmart and Target, to develop internal chemical policies banning the most common and hazardous chemicals (such as certain flame retardants and BPA) from many of the products on their shelves, including their own store brands. But beauty retailers such as Sephora and Ulta weren't having even basic conversations about toxic chemicals in products at this point. It was clear that the sector could benefit from people on the inside pushing for change. So when a few weeks later I was offered the job, I said yes.

After work one evening, Andy and I grabbed dinner at a quiet restaurant and I tearfully gave him my notice. It was one of the harder conversations I've ever had, and given the job intensity and shared history we had for over five years, I appreciated the dark lighting, which made me feel a little safer in an otherwise vulnerable conversation. He didn't take the news well, pausing for a long time after I spoke. With a shaky voice and watery eyes, he asked me what he could do to get me to stay, even offering me his job.

With a heavy heart, I told him that I had made up my mind, that it was time to see if it was possible to do this work with a brand. We both knew this would be far from the last time we'd speak, given the close friendship we'd formed. Eventually Andy came around and agreed that this was the right next step in my career. He promised to mentor me as I stepped into the position of key strategist for cosmetics reform, a role he had inhabited in TSCA reform for decades. I knew virtually no one at the FDA, the government watchdog tasked with cosmetics oversight, and would lean heavily on Andy to help build my contact list.

I convinced my boyfriend of the past few years to move to the West Coast, and he headed out early to find an apartment. Once again, I found myself moving across the country with just two duffle bags in tow. My boyfriend picked me up at the airport and was quiet and awkward when I hopped in the car. I knew something was off. Rather than having an excited conversation about the next chapter and living a dreamy SoCal life, our ride was silent. I learned why upon arriving at my new apartment.

Sitting on the old carpet of a furnitureless, decrepit West Side apartment, he proceeded to break up with me, saying something I barely remember about "needing space" and "going our separate ways." I was blindsided, to say the least. I walked by myself to get some crappy strip mall takeout food and mull over the conversation. It seemed that I was going to be learning a new city of thirteen million people on my own. Welcome to LA!

On Monday morning, after a long and awkward weekend of curling up in a single sleeping bag in the bedroom—he was across the hall on the floor of the second bedroom—I pulled out a crumpled outfit from my duffle bag, hopped on my bike, and pedaled a couple of miles to my new office for my first day of work. Everyone else drove.

I was shown to my desk, positioned across from a bubbly woman who was the head of PR and quite possibly the polar opposite of me in every way. I'm pretty sure she ironed her designer jeans before heading to work. She floated through the office with confidence in her Gucci loafers, and she loved to talk. I forced my best smile and sat down at my desk, adjusting the monitor to block her face and avoid the invitation to chat. I suspected that she was the type to ask if I was dating anyone, a sore subject.

I spent most of that first week processing the unexpected breakup, crying in the bathroom stall, and then stuffing those feelings deep inside like the good Midwesterner I was. I listened in as my new colleagues talked about Mariah Carey's husband (she was married?), niche linen and tablecloth companies (this was trendy?), and who was winning the *Bachelor* pool (it aired last night?). The last five years in DC had turned me into a full-on political nerd, and I knew better now than to bring up a PBS *NewsHour* feature on well installations in Sudan. Not my audience. (Plot twist: I now count many of these Beautycounter staffers, including the chatty

PR woman, among my closest friends, and I happily discovered that some of them did in fact watch PBS. You'd think Sweater Woman would have taught me to never again judge a person by their style choices, but some lessons you have to learn twice.)

Along with getting up to speed on celebrity gossip, I was taught how to apply a smoky eye by Christy Coleman, our on-staff celebrity makeup artist with a client list that included the likes of Heidi Klum. Picking up my tiny iPhone 2 (the larger iPhone 6 had just hit the market, and nearly all my colleagues had gotten that memo), I texted my sister on the microscopic touchpad: "Not sure what I got myself into."

Despite feeling like a fish out of water in the office, I was starting to like the West Coast. I was in my early thirties, and being newly single in a warm climate, far away from the DC grind, was invigorating. I drove up the Pacific Coast Highway on the weekend, enjoyed the trendiest hand rolls in downtown LA, and spent hours at the beach reading books. I relished my weekend downtime, which allowed me to arrive on Monday morning ready to keep pace with the steep learning curve of corporate culture.

I was also starting to like the cutting-edge vibe of LA, a city that, while totally different from nerdy DC, was at the forefront of socially minded startups like Beautycounter and Alba's Honest Company. Manufacturing for eco-friendly laundry detergents was heavily centralized in Southern California, and online delivery subscription companies for healthy lifestyle products, like Thrive Market and Ritual (a supplement company—and my future employer), were scaling. Probiotic fizzy drinks populated boutique and big-box stores alike, and sustainable fashion brands like Patagonia, Allbirds, and MATE the Label were mainstreaming. The wellness industry was officially on the map and entering a massive growth spurt. It was an energetic, buzzy time to be working at one of the companies taking a stand for good, and from my new perch at Beautycounter, the possibilities seemed endless for using one of my superpowers: arming people with the right information to shop the market. Always up for a good challenge, I had no idea how hard or complicated that would become.

Combating misleading but legal marketing claims and educating consumers on the issues would become core strategies for Beautycounter, which clearly stated that nothing is chemical free and not all chemicals are toxic.

The beauty industry was built using unregulated terms like "dermatologist tested" and "pharmaceutical grade," so the influx of new terms such as "natural," "eco-friendly," "clean," "preservative free," and "nontoxic" was simply an extension of the industry's marketing playbook. Several brands tried to be conscientious in their use of descriptors, but many more did not. There was no denying the power of using this terminology from a marketing lens: the clean beauty market would soon outpace conventional beauty sales four times over. (The category is expected to hit nearly $40 billion in US sales by 2033.)

Taking a science-first approach to brand communications, Beautycounter made its mark as one of the trustworthy players by talking about the "Never List": the ingredients that Beautycounter would intentionally not use in its formulas. The list started with 1,500 banned ingredients (it was up to 2,800 by the time I left) that solid research had found were questionable, combined with regulatory lists like those used in the EU. This early work to educate the market about how some (but not all) ingredients used in beauty products had dubious health effects wasn't easy. Any marketer would tell you that wasting a lot of time and copy talking about what's not in your product isn't a great strategy. But for us, it was a requirement and an essential part of our advocacy goals, since so few people know about the safety issues in the beauty industry.

The key was to trust that the consumer could handle a little more detail than simply "avoid this." On our website, in our marketing materials, and in the training of our saleswomen who sold directly to consumers, we explained the science that played a role in our decisions and stressed the lack of safety regulations.

It was a fine line to walk, and not all brands were as careful as Beautycounter in their approach. Many other beauty company founders were inspired by the Never List and started touting their own lists of restricted ingredients, but they provided less explanation of the complicated science and made zero reference to the dismal state of beauty regulation in our country. Some clean beauty brands went too far, relying only on messaging intended to scare people into avoiding anything with a synthetic chemical.

Retailers like Sephora and Ulta eventually developed their own lists and certifications, a huge signal that clean products were important to consumers and weren't going away. Though promising at the outset, some of these beauty retailer programs set a low bar. Most clean beauty brands today simply rely on retailer requirements, which (with the exception of Credo) are easy to achieve considering they don't require comprehensive safety testing and ban a relatively small list of ingredients (compared to the two thousand-plus that Beautycounter banned). The watered-down version of "clean" shortchanges the real work to make products safer and fails to push brands to screen ingredients for safety (looking at health endpoints like cancer, reproductive toxicity, and harm to the developing brain). What goes *into* our products is more important than what is left *out*, after all.

With all of these complexities, including the jungle of marketing terms, the question for consumers quickly became: Who was legit when formulating clean? And who was simply using a fear of chemicals as a marketing tactic?

In trying to answer this question for consumers, I quickly learned that banning ingredients was the easy part; making a product with ingredients carefully screened for hazards and reducing the risk of hidden contaminants was where the hard work lay and separated the faux clean brands from the real deals.

Sitting with the Beautycounter team early on in my tenure, I was surprised to discover the reason for our top-of-the-morning meeting: we were going to have to completely ditch our new formulas for blush, eye shadow, lipstick, and tinted moisturizer, all of which were slated to round out the skin and body care offerings already in the market.

"We got the test results back, and the levels of heavy metals are through the roof, far exceeding our internal limits," my colleague shared. "We need to start from scratch." The team let out a collective sigh.

The hypothesis was that our use of only natural pigments when we designed the first formulas contributed to the high levels of heavy metals. Natural pigments, it turned out, are sometimes higher in heavy metal contamination compared to their synthetic counterparts, since heavy metals such as lead, cadmium, and arsenic are naturally occurring in the Earth's crust. I was floored. Despite being in the know, I thought that the "natural" makeup brands, like the ones I'd been buying at Whole Foods for years, were inherently safer, that they would be delivering fewer heavy metals onto my lips with a swipe of "rosebud red" or "princess pink." Not so.

Another inadvertent misstep: we'd been intentionally formulating blushes and eye shadows without talc, a natural substance used in the base of most pressed powder cosmetics that research (some of it conflicting) had found concerning links to cancer (occupational exposure was correlated with lung cancer) and possibly increased the risk of cervical cancer (it is classified as "probably carcinogenic" when applied in the genital region on babies and adults). But skipping the talc was raising the overall percentage of natural pigment in the product, and therefore the heavy metal content.

I sat there taking in the information.

In making key ingredient decisions to manufacture safer cosmetics, we'd embraced a "better safe than sorry" approach (called the "precautionary principle"), but in this unique instance, that approach actually ended up making our products riskier. I thought about the market that Beautycounter was now playing in, which was mostly focused on "natural as safer," and wondered how many other companies made the same assumptions but never tested for heavy metals.

When we commissioned our own testing of those competitors to find out, we discovered that nearly all of the natural brands on the market had higher levels of heavy metals, like lead, cadmium, and arsenic, than the conventional brands. It was a stunning revelation. Turns out, makeup is an inherently dirty business. It was also clear that there was no part of developing clean makeup that would be easy. We went back to the drawing board and came up with a safer mix of synthetic and natural colorants. We also implemented an industry-leading program: testing every batch of color cosmetics before it went to market.

As the years passed, so too did my scope and role within the business. Although I was hired exclusively to lead advocacy, I started taking over the safety and testing department, along with packaging, responsible sourcing, and quality assurance. I went from sitting in on meetings, absorbing the information, to being in the driver's seat, a very challenging position in which I had to operationalize safety and deliver products to the market that met our own high standards. The reality was that the FDA's narrow guidance and oversight on ingredients in makeup did very little to protect human health. Case in point: the voluntary limit (read: a mere suggestion for companies) for lead in cosmetics is ten parts per million, which is very high when you consider the federal drinking water limit is a much more aggressive fifteen parts per billion. (Even though these are different routes of exposure—dermal versus ingestion [an important caveat]—the difference in limits is still stark considering the scientific community states that there is no safe level of lead.)

All this new intel had me doing some Monday morning quarterbacking on my time as a lobbyist. I would often scoff when someone told me, "Eighteen months isn't long enough to reformulate our lotion without X or Y," thinking it was a BS cover for companies to slow-walk the removal of a toxic chemical. Now I realized that some (but not all) of the product shaming I'd done wasn't fully warranted, because the entire supply chain—from raw materials to manufacturing to packaging—was open to unintentional contamination by some of the most problematic chemicals.

Take our old friend PFAS, also on the Never List. Even if a company intentionally avoided using PFAS, it might very well end up there anyways. Gulp. From the PFAS coating on the paddles used to mix color cosmetics in a steel drum to the phthalate-leaching plastic tubing used in manufacturing equipment, there are many routes of unintentional contamination. Things weren't as clear-cut as I had hoped, and like most consumers, I had assumed that companies have more control over their production than they actually do. (If you're thinking, "Well, why don't companies just build their own manufacturing facility?"—great question—the fact is that for 99 percent of companies it doesn't make financial sense, nor is it sustainable for every company to erect its own facility. So contracted manufacturing is the way the majority of beauty products are made.)

Supply chain contamination is one reason why banning a toxic chemical at the federal level is the best fix, period. Not only that, but without federal regulation, there is no incentive for suppliers to do their due diligence—to vet and to test. A clean company could ask its ingredient supplier, "Is this red pigment treated with PFAS?" (PFAS can be used to help make color cosmetics "long wear"), and many suppliers would hand them a piece of paper that says they "did not intentionally add PFAS." But they are not required to test for it or to ask their supplier that question.

On Beautycounter's Never List was another great example of the challenges we faced: formaldehyde and formaldehyde-releasing ingredients, which at the time were commonly used to help preserve personal care products. (Reminder: formaldehyde is a known human carcinogen and potent skin allergen.) Despite being a banned ingredient, formaldehyde could sneak into finished products through the packaging. Take skin serums, which feature specialized pumps: inside those pumps are various materials, including springs and plastics, such as polyoxymethylene (POM), which is made with formaldehyde and is therefore notorious for leaching formaldehyde, unintentionally contaminating products. So the formula inside the bottle could be clean, but once it passes through a pump that releases tiny amounts of formaldehyde, the lotion or serum is carrying toxic hitchhikers.

Traditional toxicologists and cosmetic chemists—who typically embrace Team Old Science—have stated in press interviews that the tiny amounts of formaldehyde from a pump won't pose any huge health risk. There is truth to that if you are considering the exposure in the total vacuum of a onetime or single-product use. However, in the real world, exposure to a chemical typically occurs multiple times via different sources over the course of a day and our entire lives. Someone dispensing skin serum daily from a formaldehyde-contaminated POM pump could also be experiencing formaldehyde exposure from their workplace, the off-gassing furniture in their home, and their nail polish or hair treatment, or as such exposure naturally occurs in an apple. (Some fruits release low levels as a by-product of metabolism, a fact that the chemical industry loves to point out as a way to make formaldehyde exposure sound safe.) The fact is that safer packaging—simple jars made from glass, aluminum, or safer plastics like polylactic acid (PLA)—has existed for years and is widely used in the market.

This is all to say that I was starting to grasp there were certain things within our control (banning formaldehyde as an intentionally used ingredient) and many things outside of our control (unseen contaminants in the supply chain, such as PFAS, phthalates, and heavy metals).

When faced with these challenges, we always turned to prominent scientists, the Shanna Swans and Arlene Blums of the world. Sprinkled throughout a week of meetings were phone calls with such trusted advisers. When it came to formulating color-rich products, we often consulted Dr. Leonardo Trasande, the same pediatrician and prominent researcher I'd asked to speak at Jessica Alba's press conference years prior, and a leader in understanding the impacts of hormone-disrupting chemicals and heavy metals on our health. Among the questions we asked: How could we make important incremental progress without promising perfection? Based on conversations with our suppliers, it was clear that very few (if any) companies had been trying to solve this problem.

I was also learning how expensive it was to create nontoxic products. Safer ingredients and packaging were often more costly, and our testing budget had to be large enough to cover costs for heavy metal testing of every batch before a product went to market. In addition, we were paying the salaries of legit scientists and PhDs on our staff, something still rare even among "clean" brands.

The higher cost of making a safer product was inevitably passed along to the consumers, at least the ones who could afford to pay it. A group of early adopters emerged to support the clean market, a cultural faction I call **the perfectionists**—wellness-obsessed urban women.

Many of these health zealots started their wellness journey through food, moving away from processed and packaged foods and toward whole foods. While that's actually a great step forward for a population addicted to processed food (Cheez-It lover here), the messaging had an air of exclusion and condescension—clearly not everyone has access to organic food, the money to buy it for their entire family, and the time to whip up truffle ricotta dip with artisan honey. (The hyperfocus on clean eating is also a way for many adherents to perpetuate a diet culture playbook of hard-and-fast rules that label noncompliance as "bad" and strict obedience as "good.") I found this group's detours away from science and their "holier than thou" attitude particularly troubling because the attention given to them tainted the entire clean movement, painting anyone who was working toward safer products as woo-woo and snobby, which was far from the truth. I knew our movement was mostly made up of people like Andrea from Iowa, and she was far from condescending. Nor was she wealthy.

The perfectionists, who were posting reels of their curated and sometimes bizarre lifestyles on social media, gave a lot of fodder to a different group, a small one at the time: **the dismissers**. They were proponents of old-school toxicology when speaking about chemical safety, and their main message was "stop fearmongering!" Dismissers were diametrically opposed to the perfectionists and took a proactive approach by trying to discredit many pillars of clean beauty and the up-to-date science underpinning it.

As I studied the early dismisser social media accounts (I was getting the sense that they were not going to go away), I noticed they were mostly reposting information from cosmetic chemists, who sound legit, being actual chemists and all, but who know very little about the safety of chemicals. Their expertise lies in mixing ingredients to make a serum, night cream, or mascara. Their accounts were essentially megaphones for the chemical industry's old talking points, namely, that we already had substantial safety regulations in place and that all this talk about toxic chemicals in our products was a marketing scam and causing undue panic.

All of it—the culture wars, the marketing BS, the never-ending pushback by the chemical industry—made my blood boil. Somewhere in the middle were the scientists, our growing Beautycounter crew of activist women, and concerned moms. This group of individuals didn't immediately react when seeing content online, and they refused to buy into simplified distillations of very complicated topics.

Left out of the conversation altogether were the communities suffering the worst consequences, the folks living where many of the toxic chemicals ended up (Arctic sinkholes, communities next to incinerators) or where they originated—the plants spewing toxic chemicals into the air and water. Many of the people in these communities weren't adding $100 creams and jade eggs to their shopping carts. They were shopping where they could afford to—at dollar stores where "bargain" products harbored the worst of the worst: oxybenzone, a problematic sunscreen ingredient linked to hormone disruption; volatile organic compounds (VOCs) in nail polish; and even the toxic metal mercury, which is intentionally used to make skin lightening creams.

The only solution that would protect the most vulnerable was policy reform: updating TSCA and the dusty 1938 cosmetic safety law would force the entire supply chain to clean up its act. Blanket regulation would make all products safer for everyone and ultimately bring down the cost of doing business the clean way. We'd already seen this drop in the cost of safer items in other product categories—toys, couches, electronics, and cleaners. Formulating clean may have been more expensive at the time, but it didn't have to be in the future. The passage of laws to remove toxic chemicals doesn't raise costs for all products and actually helps drive down costs for the whole market.

For this reason, Beautycounter consistently invested in lobbying efforts, starting with educating the people selling our growing arsenal of clean beauty products and, in turn, our customers. Slowly but surely, we found ways to translate the most important aspects of the beauty business into activism. I understood that informing laypeople about the complicated nuances could be overwhelming; most people just wanted to shop quickly for a new serum or shade of lip gloss. But I knew I also had to make them understand and care about the federal policy changes we needed. The idea was that we weren't just making and selling better, safer products, but using lipstick and lotion as a delivery system for sexy advocacy.

Several times a month we'd hold training sessions for our company's growing network of salespeople, women who weren't all that different from the moms who walked alongside me in our DC stroller brigades. These women were a drop more savvy about the marketplace, but none of them would identify as "activists," a label that carried a negative association with bandana-wearing, bare-faced, scruffy people holding signs and shouting (raises hand). Still, I was heartened to see that they seemed as excited about advocacy as they did about selling products. So I followed my tried-and-true blueprint to turn them from salesperson into activist, starting with the basics:

"We can all agree that banning smoking on airplanes was a good thing, right? That having limits on alcohol and requiring infant car seats were the smart moves? That removing lead from gasoline so fumes at the pump didn't lead to brain damage was common sense?" No argument there.

"Those lifesaving laws took time and effort to get passed. This is no different. We have as much good science telling us these chemicals are harming us as we had with cigarettes and drunk driving accidents." Translation: We had to give as much of a shit about what was going into a lipstick as we did about how that lipstick made us look.

I also explained that we needed to tackle both TSCA and the law specific to the beauty industry, FDCA. I then went back to one of my most effective tools—storytelling—and shared the disturbing tale behind the origin of the FDCA. Not surprisingly, I told them, several key women were the engines driving progress.

In 1933, a woman in Dayton, Ohio, Mrs. Brown, was being honored by her local PTA and decided to treat herself to a makeover at her local beauty salon beforehand. Her stylist suggested she take it up a notch and use a newer product called Lash Lure, which tinted eyelashes so that users wouldn't have to apply mascara every day. (At the time mascara was clumpy and easily flaked off.)

As she drove home, eager to get dressed for the ceremony, she noticed a burning sensation in her eyes and started to feel sick. Hours later, with watery swollen eyes, it was clear that Mrs. Brown wasn't heading anywhere except the hospital—something was terribly wrong. Doctors were unable to reverse the damage and several days later she was declared blind. Writing a letter to the newly formed FDA, Mrs. Brown shared her story and pleaded for them to investigate the safety of the ingredients used in salons, sharing the personal details and photos of the devastating impacts of Lash Lure. Turns out, Mrs. Brown wasn't alone—an FDA investigation found that the treatment was linked to blinding several other people and even a few deaths.

One of the officials looped into these beauty-related calamities was Ruth deForest Lamb, the FDA's chief education officer. From her perch, she was seeing a big trend in unsafe consumer products and, to put it simply, she was tired of the bullshit. She knew that while lawmakers might not respond to facts, they would respond to bad publicity. So together with FDA Chief Inspector George Lyric, Lamb created a traveling exhibit that highlighted all the horrible ways in which consumer products were harming people. (Road shows were the streaming shows of the 1930s.) The exhibit featured dangerous unlabeled ingredients and tainted products and shared horror stories like Mrs. Brown's—including pictures of her before and after the chemical chewed away her eyes.

When the road show landed at the Chicago World's Fair in 1933, a reporter dubbed the exhibit "The Chamber of Horrors." The exhibit was so effective that, after viewing it, Eleanor Roosevelt put pressure on her husband, President Franklin D. Roosevelt, and Congress to pass what became known as the Food, Drug, and Cosmetic Act of 1938. The law formally gave the FDA jurisdiction over cosmetic safety and banned eleven ingredients, including mercury.

Sort of.

The fine print: the law didn't actually ban mercury or any of the other ten ingredients, but just created an allowable level in cosmetics. Mercury's legal limit? A whopping sixty-five parts per million. To put this into perspective, the EPA's limit for mercury in drinking water is two parts per billion.

As for the poisonous ingredient in Lash Lure, it was identified as p-phenylenediamine—also known as coal tar—and was banned from use in products used on the face. But (drum roll please) this same ingredient is still legally allowed and widely used in most dark hair dyes today and linked to skin and eye irritation and cancer. Although Mrs. Brown's experience forced a key moment in the passage of the original 1938 cosmetic safety law, the reality is that the law, while well intended, wasn't written in a way that would effectively protect Americans or keep pace with what would become a fast-growing beauty market.

And alarmingly, the 1938 law failed to give the FDA the power to deem ingredients safe or unsafe; nor did it allow the agency to recall unsafe products. I would often share two examples from the last decade to underscore how dangerously weak our laws were: the FDA had tried and been unable to remove children's makeup contaminated with asbestos, nor had it been able to ban popular hair products (Deva Curl and Wen Conditioner) whose use resulted in permanent baldness. Sitting on the edges of their seats as they learned about the insane reality that makeup sold in the late 2010s was really no more regulated than in 1938, I could see these groups of women slowly becoming accidental activists.

I then closed with the surprisingly simple steps anyone can take. An action that has more impact than most people know is calling or emailing your representative. "It only takes ten calls per week on a topic for a member of Congress to pay attention to an issue," I shared, adding that every communication—email or call—is recorded as a matter of law. I also emphasized that those beta-version-looking contact forms, which live on the websites of all 435 members of Congress, were a direct line to the staffers we were lobbying. "Those messages you send from their websites land in the inbox of the very person whom we will lobby when we go to DC."

The more they talked to their friends about the incredibly ineffectual state of our federal beauty laws, the more the business and its army of saleswomen grew. Who would have guessed that the same public policy lessons we learned in middle school civics class would help a business grow in customers and revenue?

The story of the sad state of beauty product safety also needed to be shared with Hill staff and members of Congress, just as we'd educated them in the early days about TSCA. We also wanted to introduce them to Beautycounter as a brand that was doing things differently and had invested in lobbying the bill in question, the Safe Cosmetics and Personal Care Products Act, the first attempt to update the ancient 1938 cosmetic safety law. The legislation, introduced by Representative Janice Schakowsky (D-IL) in 2013, was our best shot at beauty product reform: it would give the FDA the power to actually make sure the products we reach for on shelves are safe; empower the agency to recall unsafe products; and require ingredient disclosure on all products, including those used in professional salons and sold online.

Early one fall day in 2015, I found myself on a plane headed to DC to kick off the rounds of lobbying. In a sense I was back to square one, but with one important difference: this time I had a CEO in tow . . . albeit several rows in front of me in business class. (I couldn't break the nonprofit habit of purchasing the cheapest ticket next to the restroom.) A few times during the flight I'd sneak up and chat with her. (Imagine me, à la *Bridesmaids*, parting the curtain that separated coach from business and appearing, Kristen Wiig–style, at Gregg's seat.) During one of these visits, Gregg asked me, "How long will it take to pass this legislation?"

I answered honestly: "Ten years, give or take."

She isn't the kind of person who wants to wait a decade to make meaningful change. "Do you ever get sick of doing these meetings over and over?" she asked.

I looked her in the eye and, "Yes, and so will you."

To her credit, Gregg was committed to doing whatever it would take, including endless rounds of meetings. A decade later, many mission-led CEOs and founders would embrace "activism," showing up for selfies in front of the Capitol, taking out full-page ads in the *New York Times*, and leveraging celebrities. Usually, that's where it stops. To this day I have yet to see a CEO who showed up as much as Gregg did when the cameras were off, doing the grunt work required to overhaul eighty-year-old legislation. The day-to-day work to lobby elected officials is far from sexy—it's a slog. But having Gregg at my side would give us a huge competitive edge. And Beautycounter's meteoric rise as a market leader would be a game changer.

8

THE POLITICIAN

WITH THE CEO CREDENTIALS OF BEAUTYCOUNTER'S Gregg Renfrew included in the invites, I was able to quickly secure higher-level meetings with key members of the House, the players we needed to sway votes. I was simultaneously energized and appalled by how different the reception was for a CEO than it was for the likes of an environmental or public health do-gooder. More staff took notes and asked questions, and the invitation to meet with the member of Congress directly was offered up quickly.

While I showed Gregg the legislative ropes—she was a quick study, and with each visit she leveled up her lobbying skills—I also learned a little more about her. My face time with Gregg was limited in the Santa Monica office, as she had back-to-back meetings and an aggressive travel schedule. Riding together in the back of the taxi in DC, I started to appreciate the price that entrepreneurs pay—literally—when getting something off the ground, even those funded by venture capital, as Gregg was. I pretended not to listen to her phone conversation but couldn't help but hear her asking the bank to wire funds from her personal account to the company in order to meet Friday's payroll. (Although I was used to the insecurity of a nonprofit salary, this was one of the first "oh shit" moments I had as I realized how precarious the first few years in the startup phase can be.)

About a year into these DC treks, we booked our most pivotal meeting: a sit-down with the very woman leading the charge for cosmetics safety in the House of Representatives, the fiery and sharp Representative Schakowsky. She was the first member of Congress—ever—to introduce beauty reform legislation, and it was her bill, the Safe Cosmetics and Personal Care Products Act, that we'd been supporting.

Schakowsky, the daughter of Jewish immigrants from Lithuania and Russia, had been interested in consumer safety since before many of my peers were in diapers. At age twenty-five, she led a fight as a grassroots organizer in Chicago to put freshness dates on products sold in the supermarket (illustrating, yet again, that these basic public health regulations we now take for granted happen only because someone—an activist, a politician, a mom—champions it). Since entering Congress in 1999, Schakowsky had been fighting for consumer safety regulation, unafraid to call out colleagues in either party who weren't acting in the public interest. She enthusiastically pushed for bipartisan collaboration on cutting-edge issues such as energy reform and defense spending transparency, and her no-BS, kitchen-table warmth cut through the cold jargon of political operators. She had an impressive track record of embracing compromise to get laws passed, most recently having championed the 2008 Consumer Product Safety Improvement Act, which included a federal ban on lead and certain phthalates in children's toys.

I'd met with Representative Schakowsky's staff when I first joined Beautycounter, but the landscape had changed considerably since then. We had now earned more proof points that we were a business worth paying attention to and that our salespeople were in earnest becoming activists; we'd already generated thousands of phone calls and emails to the Hill. The rapid success of Gregg's venture and other startups showed that the entire clean market had clearly taken off and wasn't just a trend, but that formulating safer products was becoming a new norm. It was time to kick everything up a notch, and joining forces with Representative Schakowsky would be key to making that happen.

While I'd lobbied Representative Schakowsky before, I'd never done so in a meeting this intimate. I was always the young kid in the back of the room, quietly observing; now I was driving the meeting. Gregg and I stepped into her office, filled with dark oak furniture, and settled onto a leather couch. (Yes, nearly every member of Congress had a leather couch—clichéd but true.) Meeting with legislative champions was always refreshing because it was less about a pitch and more about a strategy conversation. They didn't need convincing.

Short in stature and all-business, Representative Schakowsky greeted us warmly. Unlike some female politicians whose uniform is platform heels and a power suit, I noted that Schakowsky opted for a colorful button-down sweater (tenured members of Congress tended to dress more casually than newer entrants, having less to prove by way of their wardrobe choices) and sensible flat leather loafers, I imagined so she could comfortably zip around congressional corridors. The pragmatic Midwesterner in me approved.

Exchanging handshakes and smiles, I introduced Gregg to Representative Schakowsky and let her know that we had been lobbying in support of her bill for years. Gregg talked about why she started Beautycounter and how our way of doing things differently had helped us jump-start and lead the clean beauty sector with company sales that had grown over 75 percent during the past year.

Schakowsky, who already understood the problem we were trying to solve, raised her eyebrows when Gregg shared our sales numbers—she seemed impressed that we'd been able to make such a mark on the business world in such a short period of time. Gregg shared, "What our growth shows is that banning harmful ingredients from personal care products isn't anti-business, it is pro-business. And it is also the future of the beauty industry." Schakowsky nodded in agreement, her dark eyes focused intently on Gregg. I felt the thrill of having played a successful matchmaker— these two powerful women were hitting it off in the best of ways.

Schakowsky told us that she loved working on issues that focused on children and consumer safety, "the basic nuts and bolts of our everyday lives." She talked about her desire to bring more transparency to the market, including tackling the labeling loopholes. Some of the worst offenders are listed only as "fragrance" on labels of store-bought beauty products, and products sold online or in professional salons required no ingredient labeling at the time.

I let her know that Beautycounter was already working on supporting a bill in the California legislature to require ingredient transparency for professional salon products that have disparate impacts on women of color, including chemical dyes, straighteners, and nail products, which commonly contain toxic chemicals that have been linked to reproductive problems and some cancers. (The eventual passage of the California bill—led by Black Women for Wellness and Breast Cancer Prevention Partners— in 2018 would help the push for the same transparency at the federal level.)

With the big stuff covered and a shared sense of resolve established, we asked Schakowsky: How could Beautycounter's saleswomen and customers and our growing business influence support her effort to clean up the nation's beauty aisles?

Her answer was clear: "Nothing will pass unless constituents' voices are loud."

She was impressed by the grassroots work we'd been doing— getting saleswomen and customers involved through phone calls, emails, and voting—and wanted us to lean in even harder, knowing that these were the actions that would break the dam. (Years later, Schakowsky would publicly share that she thought Gregg should be the one to run for Congress. She had seen how effectively Gregg, as a businesswoman, was able to mobilize tens of thousands of women around a bipartisan cause; the network of salespeople for Beautycounter would reach over 50,000.)

Schakowsky closed the meeting by asking that we speak with her colleagues on the Energy and Commerce Committee as soon as possible so that, as she continued drumming up support, especially with her Republican counterpoints, they'd be primed. She understood that it would be a different conversation now that businesses like ours had proven it was possible to do two things at once: manufacture products the market desired while also making them safer.

I told her we'd do just that and felt a surge of excitement and pride that we were partnering with the likes of Schakowsky. I could tell Gregg was pumped too.

We left Schakowsky's office recharged for this next phase in the fight. Gregg and I would need that energy for the long two-day lobby sprint I had planned for us—back-to-back meetings and thousands of steps clocked each day. I crammed in as many high-level meetings as possible when I had Gregg in tow. Wrapping up our most successful trip to date, it was clear that we were making progress in pushing this bill to a congressional hearing, the next phase of the legislative process.

As we sat in Gregg's hotel room that evening, with our sore feet propped up and two mediocre room service meals still on their trays, we schemed about the next step. I had my sights set on doing an en masse lobbying trip to Washington, just like the stroller brigade I'd organized years earlier in DC. This type of trip for a consumer brand was unheard of at the time.

"We now have a critical mass of informed women, but this time instead of pushing strollers, these women will be wielding lipstick," I told Gregg excitedly. When she interjected, "Safer lipstick," I smiled. "Yes, safer lipstick."

Alongside planning Beautycounter's first big group lobby trip to DC, I was also traveling to other parts of the country to help build the growing presence of Beautycounter sales advocates in key states. At times I felt like an orchestra conductor cuing the wind and string sections in the buildup to the final movement of a symphony—in this case, federal reform.

It was during one of these state trips that my nonexistent personal life took a turn for the better. A male colleague from my TSCA lobbying days reached out to see if I would help garner support for a bill he was working on in Oregon; that bill would ban sixty-six toxic chemicals from kids' products, including creams and shampoos. He was handsome, always professional, and very easy to talk to, and I quickly called him back. He asked me if I could organize Beautycounter sales reps to drive phone calls and show up for legislative hearings. I immediately said yes. He was a babe and I also wanted to show Gregg what victory felt like. Getting people to turn out for state legislative battles was a cinch compared to funneling supporters to DC for federal change, and I knew our involvement in Oregon would make a difference. These state wins were critically important to putting pressure on Congress, and participating in the Oregon initiative would also show the Beautycounter community that progress was possible. It's one thing to tell people that their voice matters—it's another to show them firsthand.

We packed the hearing rooms with our sales reps and organized a massive phone call campaign. I also testified in support of the bill, resurrecting my testimonial skills—I was no longer that anxious twenty-two-year-old whose voice shook and who worried about her credentials, although I was a little nervous with my unexpected crush sitting behind me in the audience.

The legislation passed. Having a fast-growing business on the side of a ban clearly helped. As for the dreamy guy who'd asked for my assistance? It was nerd love at its finest. We long-distance-dated, bonding over our passion for leaving the world a little better than we found it, and found relief in a shared understanding of the challenges when we downloaded the stresses of our workdays. We enjoyed weekends at the beach and ate our way around Portland, and eventually he moved to LA, where we eloped at the Beverly Hills courthouse.

On the professional front, the Oregon victory was the perfect prelude for getting our team pumped up for the big DC lobby trip that Gregg and I had hatched. We decided to hold a contest for our salespeople, but instead of using outdated sales incentives like "win the keys to a new car!," we'd offer a more experiential (and strategic) prize: the top leaders from each state would win a trip to DC to lobby Congress. We hoped that the incentives—a behind-the-scenes lobbying experience, meetings with elected officials, and personalized training from leading scientists—would fuel a healthy competition.

This contest turned out to be our most popular contest to date, and it showed me that many people really do want to be involved in their government and just need someone to show them the ropes and prove to them that it makes a difference. When the final list of one hundred women, from all fifty states, was ready, I got to work booking meetings. Lots of meetings—we ended up having 103 in one day. We asked everyone to wear the same signature red lipstick (Beautycounter Red), and I ordered gold "B" pins for us all to wear; these were a classy upgrade, I thought, from my "No More Toxic Toys" pin days. But when the pins arrived at the DC hotel the day before our lobbying meetings, I cringed: the "B" was much larger than anyone, including myself, had expected. B stood for Big apparently.

Gregg walked into the windowless conference room in the hotel basement for our morning training, laid eyes on the giant Bs, and whispered to me out of the side of her mouth that the pins were surprisingly large. Despite agreeing with her, I assured Gregg, "It will create buzz. Trust me on this one."

By the end of the day on the Hill, staff would smile as we passed them in the hall, and security guards said, "Hey, Beautycounter!" when they checked in our group, clearly identified by our hard-to-miss letter pins.

Despite representing a beauty brand, the trip wasn't about looking good. We spent time educating our grassroots Beautycounter lobbyists on how to engage in nonpartisan lobbying, and we brought in leading scientists to help them understand the complexities of the science. Among these experts were Dr. Robin Dodson, a chemical exposure researcher from the Silent Spring Institute, and Dr. Kim Harley, a reproductive endocrinologist from Berkeley. We reminded our lobbyists to say "linked to" instead of "caused" when speaking about the health impacts of chemicals and to convey that not all chemicals were toxic, that certain chemical preservatives, for example, were a key part of a winning clean formula. This lobbying effort was not about ridding products of all chemicals, but rather eliminating the intentional use of unsafe ones.

Despite our varying political views, we were united as a group through our shared cause. It was refreshing to find community without the negativity. As the world increasingly became more partisan, these in-person moments, centered on an issue we all cared deeply about, were a potent reminder of the humanity we shared.

There was Margie,* a woman with long wavy auburn hair from Kentucky. She shared with me that she and her husband went to the same country club as one of their senators, who also happened to be a key Republican whose support we wanted to garner. They supported his political campaigns and even spent time socially with him and his kids, and she agreed to help us get a meeting with him. (Seeing that one of his voters, and a friendly face at that, was lobbying in person made it clear to the senator that the bill was not the result of partisan politics.)

Another one of our saleswomen trainees was a model from Georgia who shared that not only did she have difficulty finding makeup artists whose kits carried shades dark enough for her skin tone, but that she also couldn't find safer full-coverage makeup for her photo shoots. Beautycounter was the only clean foundation that worked with her deep skin tone.

The arbitrary political walls erected by ideological establishments, politically charged TV networks, and elected officials themselves quickly crumbled as we pushed forward with our group of women.

---

* Name has been changed to protect identity.

Sitting down for dinner, after a long day on the Hill, at a hotel restaurant overlooking the White House, you could feel the shared connection, warmth, and energy in the room as we clinked our wineglasses and took selfies. Later I glanced across the room and locked eyes with Gregg, who mouthed to me, "Thank you."

Just a month after this trip, sitting in Santa Monica at my sun-splashed desk one afternoon, I called Andy to ask for his advice on how to handle a few of the thornier policy topics, like how ingredient suppliers were currently let off the hook for safety when we knew they were also part of the problem.

He interrupted me. "Lindsay, stop."

He was unusually abrupt, so I froze midsentence.

"A small group is putting the finishing touches on the final TSCA bill. We expect it to come up for a final vote in a week," he said.

Normally not particularly expressive, I felt my jaw drop as I clutched my cell phone. I was silent for a beat and then asked the million-dollar question: "How strong is the final bill?"

Before any bill went up for a vote, negotiations inevitably watered things down. Compromise is the only way any major reforms happen—as Schakowsky had also emphasized in our meeting—and I wanted to know what Andy and team had been able to save. He launched into a rundown of the wins in the bill and some of what was left out. I put down the phone and sat back in my chair. I couldn't believe it. Years of lobbying efforts for federal reform, from all corners, had finally paid off.

In a Rose Garden signing ceremony in June 2016, a few weeks after our conversation, President Barack Obama signed into law important updates to TSCA. Most notably, the bill strengthened the safety standard (a term used to define how a chemical is determined to be "safe"). It also replaced the cost-benefit loophole with one that used a health standard to determine whether a toxic chemical should be pulled from the market—a giant win. (Reminder: In 1989, under the old cost-benefit safety standard, the EPA had tried to ban asbestos and failed.) And the law gave the EPA enhanced authority to review and test new and existing chemicals. What it didn't do: fund safer chemistry innovation, provide explicit protections for fenceline communities, or ban the worst chemicals, like PBTs or PFAS; and in certain instances it hindered state lawmakers' ability to pass new strong laws.

Imperfect as the final bill was, it was the culmination of decades of incredibly hard work. We celebrated the TSCA win within the Beautycounter community through a happy hour for the staff and shared the good news online with the salespeople.

I hoped capitalizing on the law's passage would keep Gregg bought into this work, but she was already sold. Pulling me into her beautiful office at the end of a long corridor, she said, "Congrats on TSCA. What's next?" I assured her I was plotting our next move to keep the momentum going. Our work was far from done.

The honest truth was that while the TSCA win was flawed in many ways, it filled my tank too, providing me with a renewed sense of hope for updating our cosmetics safety laws. Although I'd long ago accepted the existential nature of this work—there was always more to do—I hadn't quite realized that after all those years of slogging away in DC, I needed the win to believe that sweeping federal reform was possible. I thought back to the first time I learned that our laws had not caught up to the alarming science, that toxic chemicals in my over-the-counter perfume were hacking my hormones, and that my niece's bath toys could be harming her fertility. One woman—Sweater Woman—had set me straight. I'd been moved to take up the fight and stake my career on the belief that if enough people knew what I knew and what the scientists knew, we could live in a safer world. It felt surreal to connect the dots from a meeting fifteen years ago with the news that a reformed TSCA had passed.

As thrilled as I was about this professional victory, I was more excited about my own new chapter: parenthood. After TSCA reform passed, I was standing in the tiny kitchen of our retro apartment building, newly married, nauseous, and holding a positive pregnancy test. My husband, who was making dinner, turned around to see me smiling and handing him the little plastic stick that foretold the story of a new, incredible, and complicated journey into parenthood. We hugged until he smelled the dinner burning on the stove.

Because we'd both spent considerable time in the field of consumer safety, the shift to prepping for baby was relatively easy for us. We knew which brands were truly flame-retardant free when shopping for a crib mattress, we could quickly decide which baby bottles were our top pick (glass), and I didn't need to look up which mercury-soaked fish to avoid while pregnant. Also absent was any pushback from my husband about the need to invest in safer products. This had been a consistent problem for moms that came up over the years: "How do I convince my husband that we need to change our laundry detergent?"

Having all of this information at the forefront of our minds—from years spent talking to parents and experts—was not lost on us. I couldn't imagine starting from scratch as a new parent, having to research all the product categories and decipher the science, build a registry, and also grow a human. The extra burden on parents to police the products on shelves was so unfair. Our resolve that policy work was the ultimate, equitable solution only grew alongside our soon-to-be firstborn daughter.

With an expanding belly, I hopped back on a plane to DC—this time solo—to pull another trick out of my hat (thanks Andy!). I would be hosting a congressional briefing, an educational event where experts fly in to bring Hill staff up to speed on certain top-ics. It's like having twenty-five to fifty Hill meetings at the same time in one big room. (At this point in the journey, I was a fan of efficiency.) Shimmying my way into a pencil skirt that was now barely closing in the back, I wore an extra-long jacket to hide my not-yet-revealed condition. I stood outside the briefing room and chatted with the experts on deck, one of whom was environmental and maternal health researcher Ami Zota from George Washington University (and now faculty at Columbia University), discussing the flow of the briefing and what to expect from the audience.

I welcomed the crowd and gave a brief overview of the clean marketplace—the good, the bad, and the ugly. I explained that there were substantial business and economic benefits to making nontoxic products for a growing consumer base hungry for them. We had much to celebrate, I said, but cautioned that there were gap-ing holes that commerce alone could not fix.

Having teed up why we were all there, I stepped aside as Zota walked up to the podium to deliver her searing remarks.

Zota was the ideal scientist to make the case for the intersec-tion between science, beauty, and social justice. Petite, with curly, dark hair and serious eyes, she silenced the room as she began her presentation, grounding us in the fact that while we were here to talk about beauty product safety, the issues at hand were larger.

"Beauty is power," she opened, pausing for a moment to look at the audience.

Continuing in an even tone, she said, "Historically, beauty has been a gendered form of power that has real social and economic benefits. Whether it's increasing your marriage potential or increas-ing your likelihood to get a certain job, these beauty norms affect all of us and especially women of color and other marginalized populations that sit outside of that norm."

It wasn't an opening the Hill staff were expecting. They looked up from their phones. Zota officially had their attention.

She continued: "One way we may adapt to achieve those beauty standards is by using more products, increasing our exposure to toxic ingredients. Which can have biological and physical consequences on our health. It is the science around those health effects that I want to share more about with you today."

Zota had codeveloped a framework through which to see beauty, a lens that she called, pointedly, the environmental injustice of beauty. "I want to shine a light on social and structural factors that impact our exposures to toxic chemicals in beauty products. What we find beautiful as a society is shaped by racism, colonialism, sexism, classism," she told the audience. "These forces," she maintained, "had direct impacts on women's exposures to toxic chemicals."

Zota studied the link between ingredients in toxic products targeted at women of color (hair relaxers with formaldehyde, douches loaded with phthalates, talcum powder with asbestos, skin lightening creams with mercury) and hormonally driven conditions (such as pregnancy complications like high blood pressure, menopause, fibroids) and cancers such as breast and uterine cancer.

The research was damning: women who are regular users of hair relaxers—which contain problematic ingredients like formaldehyde, certain parabens, phthalates, and cyclosiloxanes—are twice as likely to develop uterine cancer compared to non-users, and Black women use relaxers more frequently than women of other racial groups. (There is some evidence that lye-based relaxers have less formaldehyde, though more research on them needs to be conducted.) Even worse, certain hair relaxer brands—like Brazilian Blowout—were found to have up to 10 percent of the formula formaldehyde.

The audience was sober, and I watched them closely. Nearly

everyone had eyes on Zota or was scribbling down notes to share with their boss. Zota closed by sharing with Hill staff the important role they played in helping solve these heavy issues. "One of the best tools we have to advance health equity is public policy, because market-based reforms are still ad hoc. The ninety-nine-cent stores are lagging behind Target, and the market alone can't solve this problem. Right now, safer products are still more expensive, but they don't have to be."

As congressional staff filed out of the briefing room, several looked me straight in the eye and shared how helpful the information was. For the first time in years, I could see the end game for beauty reform. Years of infrastructure had been built, and a steady drumbeat of people from all over the country were emailing and calling Congress about the need for updated beauty laws. The passage of a reformed TSCA had also shown that consumer safety legislation was popular with various constituencies across the United States.

Hill staff were more engaged than ever, and the list of state consumer safety laws was getting longer. By this point, Beautycounter's efforts—amplifying the work of leading nonprofits—had helped pass over a dozen state clean beauty laws. (The tally would be over fifteen by the time I left.) In California and New York, new ingredient disclosures became mandatory for professional products in salons—an important regulation given that research has shown that nail technicians suffer miscarriages at a much higher rate than the rest of the population. We also helped pass a landmark ban on certain PFAS chemicals in cosmetics sold in California and a federal green chemistry incentive to encourage companies to make safer ingredients.

And thanks to several years of lobbying and testifying in Washington State by Zota, Toxic Free Future, and Representative Sharlett Mena, we helped pass the strongest state bill restricting toxic chemicals in beauty products. Each bill passing had brought us one step closer to updating those 1938 federal beauty laws, creating the pressure on Congress that it could no longer ignore.

On Christmas Day in 2018, we welcomed our daughter into the world, and my relationship with this work would no longer be the same. I was now grappling with a deeper drive, a fierce evolutionary desire to fight for and protect the world that my little girl was going to grow up in. Specifically, I thought about "future generations," a phrase I had used for years but was now thinking about differently: "If she wanted to start a family, what would the world be like for her child?"

My maternity leave quickly faded behind me, and I reentered the fray, picking up where I left off. I no longer harbored a shred of doubt about whether my decision to switch to the industry side would make a difference. (I patted my younger self on the back for that giant leap of faith.) We were galvanizing thousands of women, controlling some of the levers behind the corporate curtain, and continuing the steady drumbeat of actions that would get us to the next phase of the legislative process: lobby, educate the grassroots, work the press. Wash, rinse, repeat. Adding to the momentum was an uptick in helpful (at the time) press coverage. Each week new headlines appeared in mainstream publications like the *Washington Post* and the *New York Times* as well as beauty-focused publications like *Allure* and *Glossy* that highlighted the science around certain chemicals used in beauty products, including instances of "buyer beware" and voluntary recalls issued by the FDA, such as recalls of dry shampoo found to contain benzene and children's makeup that harbored asbestos.

While I found it was sometimes risky to speak to the press—I never knew their true angle and whether they would take a quote out of context—the people writing about these topics were becoming increasingly savvy and (mostly) able to accurately translate the important research into digestible and usable information for readers. The crescendo was growing.

Early one morning in the spring of 2020, I was playing with my daughter on the floor, wearing my work clothes and drinking coffee as we batted a ball back and forth. She smiled and giggled, and I looked at the clock, trying to stay present for the few minutes I had with her before being gone all day in the office. I was distracted, thinking about a press interview I had scheduled later that morning with a reporter covering some of the state clean beauty bills that were passing.

When our caregiver arrived, I kissed my daughter on the top of her head, hopped on my bike, and rode down the palm tree–lined streets. I didn't know that it was the last morning I would follow this routine. Later that afternoon our office shut down for "two weeks" because of an emerging global virus we all knew very little about. Sitting down at my desk, I did the interview and learned that the story would run the following day. I prepped the team, letting them know we would have a press story to help share and celebrate the new policy wins with our community.

The collective Beautycounter community now numbered over 50,000, and their posts and customers reached millions of North Americans. Every news article, every social media post, every "like" from a friend was fuel for all of us as we entered the next and final phases of the battle. We were continuing to push for bills in both the House and Senate aimed at fixing the core elements of the broken 1938 law: allowing the FDA to assess ingredients for safety (and in some cases ban the worst offenders); enabling the FDA to recall harmful products (like children's makeup with asbestos or the popular shampoo linked to permanent baldness); closing the fragrance loophole; and increasing transparency for ingredients used by salon professionals.

But along with all those helpful posts and likes and tweets, I was becoming increasingly aware of the dark side of social and traditional media. Interspersed among the high-fives in the DMs of my personal social handles were messages from our saleswomen alerting me to accounts and news stories that were misstating important information, either through fearmongering or by dismissing strong science. Those early adopters—the perfectionists—were "doing their own research" and veering into dicey territory, blending content around the need to remove PFAS from cosmetics (great) with questionable content, like curing your kids' colds by putting sliced onions on the bottoms of their feet (there's no science behind this technique) and not wearing sunscreen because, they claimed, all sunscreens give you cancer (just . . . nope). And the cosmetic chemists, who were feeding off of this more egregious content easily and rightly rebuffing old wives' tales and extreme takes on sun protection, were also dismissing the legit science-backed messages, claiming that "phthalates in cosmetics are not disrupting your hormones" and "all sunscreens are safe." In the frenzied and anything-goes climate of social media, the cosmetic chemists seemed like the level-headed group and built substantial followings by telling everyone to "calm down, nothing to see here, folks."

Instagram had become a helpful tool I used to quickly fact-check misinformation, but the inaccuracies were spreading quickly, even from people who meant well. "Friendly note, natural beauty products aren't automatically safer!" I typed on one popular influencer's comment section, then logged off so I could get to my never-ending legislative call list and not get sucked into what were sure to be dozens of replies to my reply.

That afternoon I rode my bike home early, due to the unforeseen office closure, and gave my daughter a big hug when I walked through the door. Hunched over and working from our bed, I drafted some social media copy in anticipation of the press story hitting the airwaves the next day.

I could hear my daughter playing peek-a-boo with my caregiver downstairs and wished I could join them. The next morning I woke up and started a work routine that would soon become the new pandemic norm: working from home and witnessing the beauty of my child's life—so much more easily than when I was at the office—along with navigating the insanity of parenting between Zoom meetings.

I walked to my annual OB appointment later that day. In the waiting room, I talked with a few other patients about the wild nature of this new global virus and how strange it was to be on day one of a "lockdown." What I kept to myself: How in the hell would I manage parenting and work and life if we couldn't keep our caregiver? Even with a supportive partner (who was also pulling long hours so we could afford our small Santa Monica rental), my days were one big blur of racing from work to home to plane and back again. Adding a pandemic to the mix? Impossible.

As I lay on the noisy crumpled paper of the exam table, I told my OB I'd been experiencing a lot of fatigue and bloating, and she ran some tests. I was looking at the bright fluorescent lights on the ceiling when she reentered the room and shared some very unexpected news: "Lindsay, you're pregnant."

9

THE INFLUENCERS

GOING FROM BEING AN ACTIVE MOM WITH A FAST-PACED job, a young baby, and a lively travel calendar to a first-trimester shut-in with a crawling toddler was . . . well, let's just say it wasn't my smoothest life transition. Because my husband and I were suddenly tag-teaming childcare while working full-time, I had to carry my fourteen-month-old while on calls to keep her from getting into dangerous situations and pulling books off shelves.

Going for long walks and constantly bouncing a baby might sound like a great way to stay in shape during a lockdown pregnancy, but as the months progressed (the "two-week" office shutdown was now a joke) and my daughter got bigger, it took a toll. One afternoon in early summer, I found I was bleeding. A lot. I raced to my OB (solo—my husband wasn't allowed to join me because of Covid restrictions), who told me that the excessive baby carrying had made part of my placenta pull off of my uterine wall. My doctor explained that as long as I stopped holding my daughter and gave up my long walks (my only form of entertainment during the lockdown), she was confident the pregnancy would be successful.

As any mom knows, this was a tall order, especially considering the unusual circumstances and my all-consuming job, but I took the OB's advice seriously. My husband stepped up to pinch-hit, and I placed my daughter on the floor next to me and handed her toys while I took Zoom meetings. The stark reality was that she too had to adapt.

Each day we all got used to what it meant to do this work in a remote environment. Happily, business was booming at Beautycounter, unlike many companies during the pandemic. We continued to grow, in part because of social media platforms like Instagram and the lesser-known TikTok, which a few of our saleswomen were starting to experiment with to tout Beautycounter's products and mission. Individuals with social media platforms were becoming more influential as people leaned heavily on technology to stay connected.

I had spent years training Beautycounter salespeople on best practices to communicate the complicated science of toxic chemicals. Some of them were formal influencers with large platforms who often promoted brands, while many others were considered "micro-influencers," with followings between 10,000 and 50,000. I also did live trainings and developed brand guidelines for talking about Beautycounter's offerings and for activism on social media, which helped get the message out quickly. Many of these women were becoming the friend people turned to for advice on topics that went beyond their training, such as which cleaning or baby products to buy, or what a headline about new research on chemicals in furniture meant for their family. These influencers then turned to me for answers. My DMs filled up daily, and I did my best to keep up with the questions. I was happy that our salespeople were trying to speak responsibly about the science and the marketplace, so despite the fact that my day job had very little to do with spending time on social channels, I worked overtime addressing the FAQs.

The run-amok nature of social media, however, was making it harder than ever to manage my inbox. I was increasingly being tagged by our salespeople in problematic posts they were stumbling across, content from popular accounts that were misstating facts, whether they knew it or not. "Lindsay, FYI this account is saying phthalates in fragrance are safe, can you weigh in?" "Heads up, she is stating that anything with natural ingredients is non-toxic!"

Seeing the little red icon indicating new messages went from an exciting dopamine hit to a moment of dread. As the polarized conversations about "clean" intensified on social media, I tried ignoring these posts. I had zero time, and I knew that more engagement would boost their algorithms. But as the months ticked by, it became harder and harder to dismiss. Social media, which we'd initially harnessed as a tool to share decades' worth of science, was quickly becoming a weapon turned against us. Along with a growing interest in safer products came the pushback (for every action there's a reaction) from influencers questioning research they didn't understand and dismissing any merit to terms like "green" and "clean." The early days of a toxicologist or wellness "expert" occasionally posting something false or fearmongering were long gone. Now the misinformation was widespread, like an out-of-control virus.

Speaking of viruses, some of the madness was directly due to the pandemic, which had ushered in an era of rapid proliferation of misinformation that fed disdain for mainstream public health recommendations. It didn't help that government and state leaders couldn't agree on guidelines. In the wake of all the confusion, individuals with huge platforms and little expertise were stepping in to direct traffic, wielding unprecedented power and spreading anti-science messages that had real impacts on people's health.

Questioning well-established science had become acceptable during the pandemic. And consumer safety and clean beauty issues were getting caught in the crosshairs.

Some doctors, scientists, and other educated groups, seeing how disinformation was being weaponized, tried to right the ship by speaking to the media and using their platforms to educate people on the facts. But there weren't nearly as many influential voices countering the BS. Also, environmental health scientists were busy doing research and weren't exactly social-media savvy.

The other reason for the massive uptick in misinformation was the cultural phenomenon that was taking place online, fed by algorithms and growing polarization in just about every aspect of our lives. The cultural factions I'd identified in the early days of social media—the perfectionists and the dismissers—had exploded in size and complexity. The perfectionists, once made up of mostly left-leaning women filming unrelatable content in their sleek renovated kitchens, had been joined by self-proclaimed "crunchy mamas," who were also amplifying a version of clean living that distorted the movement's mission. And by "crunchy mama" I don't mean a politically progressive environmentalist that may come to mind. The term has been somewhat rebranded to describe a new melding of liberal hippies with far-right anti-government libertarians; today many "crunchy mamas" can be deeply religious, early adopters of wellness trends (including fringe things like drinking cow's colostrum), and very skeptical about science, which fuels a propensity to dabble in conspiracy theories. This group shared posts claiming that all chemicals are bad and that the "chemtrails" behind airplanes are toxic chemicals intended to intentionally sicken or mind-control populations so that Big Pharma can sell us more pharmaceuticals. (They are actually called "contrails" and are vapor streams from jet fuel that crystallize in high humidity.)

With a worldview grounded in beliefs that often don't require credible substantiation, the crunchy mama is susceptible to faux news channels that disseminate information with little scientific rigor. She tends to dismiss mainstream media, embrace dissent for societal compliance, and shun government. (The activist in me embraces some dissension, but as you can see from this book, I believe that dissenting responsibly is more complicated than criticizing everything that comes from the government or entirely accepting information from a single media channel.) Added to the online mix of cultural factions were the wellness gurus and yogis who preached the benefits of oil pulling (despite the lack of any science behind this form of dental hygiene) and shunned any form of sugar (including natural sugars present, for example, in bananas and sweet potatoes).

Watching all these subgroups merge into a convoluted demographic that ultimately shared one of the same goals I had—fewer toxic products—was disturbing. The political scientist in me found this big-tent group fascinating, but the grassroots organizer in me found it terrifying. The crunchy mamas leaned more conservative, and the urban wellness mamas trended liberal, but they had one thing in common: both groups were selling a version of clean living that didn't line up with the science. To be clear, I've always deeply believed there is space for everyone—libertarians, ultraconservatives, and uber-progressives—in the consumer safety movement. That belief still holds true today. But during the pandemic, an already nuanced topic was made exponentially more complex.

As if that wasn't enough, during this Twilight Zone moment, the influence of the dismissers—the group rallying behind Team Old Science—grew as well. They had ramped up their content, producing reels, stories, and podcasts in which they insisted that virtually all chemical safety concerns were overblown. And they had a lot of fodder.

Cosmetic chemists were now joined by dermatologists (whose field is focused mostly on efficacy and who tend to have little background in environmental health science) and science education accounts mainly featuring PhDs who worked on immunology and vaccine safety—a very different field of science in which the Shanna Swans work. As their posts received lots of comments and likes, they were incentivized to keep creating similar high-performing content. Strategically, they shared each other's posts, amplifying the reach. Every time I was tagged in these posts, my audience asking me to weigh in, I cringed at the creepily familiar talking points: they echoed the same messages I heard while sitting across from the chemical industry in tense hearings back in Minnesota or lobbying in DC.

Watching these two extreme groups feed off each other and lure thousands of followers to the outer limits, like Pied Pipers, angered and scared me. I became more convinced than ever that the solution lay in the center, in pulling away from the all-or-nothing thinking. I knew the middle was where people could focus on the facts and where we could build a meaningful base to make real progress. The lobbyist side of me was also thinking about the cultural climate in which the beauty product reform bill could have its best shot, where politicians could be tipped one way or the other based on where their constituents were at.

I knew I could cut through the noise only by meeting my audience where they were: in the digital space. And because I couldn't snuff out every fire on every irresponsible influencer's account, I spruced up my long-forgotten personal website and devoted my evening hours (I should say "hour" singular, because that's all I could steal away from mommy-ing and sleeping) to a series of blogs intended to dispel the biggest myths and target emerging cultural groups that were perpetuating dangerous misinformation.

I toiled away in the wee hours, fortifying this middle-lane cultural camp—which I'd started calling **the pragmatists**, a moderate, fact-informed faction between the two extremes—to serve as immunization against the growing army of dismissers and perfectionists, who were becoming increasingly dogmatic.

With this commonsense "we're all in this together" approach, I was also trying to counter the increasingly nasty partisan fights playing out. As someone who'd had a front-row seat to the vicious political fighting in state and federal government, I'd always taken solace in the fact that the electorate—the constituents—had a more humane and balanced approach to political conversations. Not anymore.

Like so many of us, when I logged on to Facebook, Twitter, and Instagram, I witnessed the intolerance, the inability to listen and discuss, and a general disdain for people who had different political views or supported different candidates. The clean community was far from immune to these behaviors, and I longed for the days when I sat down and pushed strollers alongside moms from all walks of life, when we knew we likely had different politics and simply didn't care because we were united on an important issue. Our experiment in supersizing a movement of beauty-minded mom activists and using corporate machinery to push reform was encountering a new Goliath—an out-of-control digital culture.

The battlefield was nasty. Friends and colleagues were lobbing insults at each other in the comments sections, including directly at me. I encountered online bullying, as did many scientists and activists I knew. A few colleagues even received threats serious enough to be reported to their superiors and the authorities. The more complex and contentious this work became, the less fun I was having.

The need to expand the pool of pragmatists seemed to grow as we got closer to the 2020 election. I continued to lean hard into the advocacy front, mobilizing the salesforce through a pragmatist's lens and passing state clean beauty laws. Educating and motivating saleswomen and consumers felt more important than ever. So did expanding our offerings and strengthening our market presence. The Beautycounter team rolled up our sleeves to launch safer versions of some of the clean beauty products that were the most challenging to make, such as mascara and anti-aging creams that would perform as well as their toxic counterparts. The world was off-balance in so many ways, but at least we'd secured a steady foothold in the market.

Still on strict orders from my doctor to skip the long walks and avoid too much activity, due to my placenta scare and "overactive uterus," I found myself working long sedentary hours in our small apartment, playing the roles I could in keeping the movement together. As I worked on building the pragmatist camp on my blog, I knew I had to get pragmatic with my own life. A few weeks before my due date, I stepped back from the fray to prioritize my physical and mental health. I put down my phone and disengaged from social media. I soaked up the remaining days as a mom to one, building and knocking down block towers with my daughter between the meetings I deemed must-attend.

On election day, November 3, my baby was four days past due, still cozy and content, so my doctor scheduled an induction. Two days later, sitting in a hospital bed and watching the election results still rolling in, I wondered what kind of world this baby would experience and how I could help make things a little less partisan, a little less ugly for her. Grateful to deliver a healthy baby girl, we headed home, me back in a diaper and mentally preparing for one of my least favorite phases of life: postpartum.

As my body slowly healed and I worked to adjust to chasing a toddler while also nursing an infant, I took a break from the online noise and gave myself a little slice of peace. When I re-engaged with work after maternity leave, I found that in those few short months, the dynamic between the extremes had gotten worse. (I hadn't thought it would get better overnight, but still . . .) Sleep-deprived and protective of my limited energy reserves, I stuck with my decision not to refute the bullshit on influencer accounts, even though followers of mine continued to tag me in the comments, hoping I'd shut them down. Instead, I looked for opportunities to reach a lot of people at once through conferences, press events, and podcasts.

In the fall of 2021, I was invited to participate in a live webinar panel to answer the question: Is clean beauty BS? It seemed like a great opportunity to channel a level-headed, nuanced perspective and speak to a broader audience. The panel was supposed to address the chasm between cosmetic chemists, who were quick to defend the use of PFAS in cosmetics (Rob Bilott and his crew would definitely disagree), and proponents of clean beauty brands, who were saying there was a grave need to make products safer.

I was thrilled to see that many beauty reporters and editors were invited. I could help dispel the tsunami of inaccuracies with this audience, the professionals whose job it was to interpret the facts for their subscribers and followers. I'd started noticing some of the beauty press parrot influencer misinformation and reshare their content, which terrified me. Several days before the event, I looked at the registration page to double-check who the other panelists were. Normally, all panelists for these types of events would do a prep call together, but the fact that no such chance to connect had been offered put me on alert.

The first panelist was, unsurprisingly, a toxicologist, an adjunct professor I'd never heard of, with no apparent background in the field of environmental health. The second panelist was a junior-level marketing person from a small clean beauty brand, a company that had no consumer safety or policy experts on staff to offer up. (Otherwise, they'd have sent someone more senior or better suited to the job.)

The third panelist was a cosmetic chemist who, like me, called herself a "science communicator," or "sci comms" for short. She was becoming quoted more often in mainstream beauty articles, and I'd been tracking her account for several years, watching her gain followers. Her posts had become more and more brazenly dismissive of decades of research showing strong links between toxic chemicals and health outcomes. She presented her online content as science-led and intended to combat fearmongering, leaning on her expertise as a formulator. While her training sounded credible to the average person, she was not an expert in chemical safety.

The tricky part was that I agreed with half of what she said. She beat the drum that "not all natural ingredients are safe and not all synthetic ingredients are toxic," a message that Beautycounter—and I personally—had been sharing for years. She also argued, rightly, that "preservative-free" as a marketing term was problematic since we needed to preserve formulas to prevent mold and bacteria from growing. I also shared this concern. But then she mixed in content that was dismissive of the science around PFAS, phthalates, and other toxic ingredients, claiming that we had nothing to fear because we were exposed to such low doses.

It was clear to me from her content that she hadn't read the pertinent studies (or didn't agree with them). Nor was she conversant in the decades of environmental health research showing that chemicals behave differently than we originally thought. The battle between old and new science was rearing its head again.

The fourth panelist was me. I realized I'd have a heavy lift in representing the research and regulation landscape, in part because my own credibility was in question—I was there representing a brand that sold products. This was one of the few moments when I missed the independence of working for the public health non-profit community.

The day of the panel I logged on, willing myself to fight the good fight. These days I had a different kind of fire in me compared to my child-free years. It wasn't that I was any more or less committed to the cause—I'd always fiercely advocated for those who couldn't advocate for themselves—but watching my little ones mouth chew toys and breathe deeply as their chubby cheeks rested on their crib mattresses, I was reminded daily of what I was fighting for. Still, that fire wasn't exactly raging. Any mom will tell you that the first year after having a baby makes you yearn for a new word to describe your exhaustion.

I'd recovered fairly quickly after my first baby, but this second birth, on top of the pandemic, had wiped me out. I thought back to all the times I'd asked moms to attend hearings and press events, and they showed up weary-bodied, with swollen breasts, carting their little ones in chest carriers and strollers. I had no idea back then of the sacrifice I was asking of them. Now I deeply understood—and was more angered than ever by the injustice of the fight continuing to fall on the shoulders of those who had the least amount of time to shop in a complicated marketplace and be politically engaged. At the toughest point in a woman's life, we are expected to also be the drivers of large-scale societal shifts.

With concealer covering deep under-eye circles, I turned on my camera and joined the panel. I was not prepared for the onslaught of misinformation and marketing spin that ensued. When I spoke about how far behind the United States was in ingredient safety compared to international markets, the cosmetic chemist pounced, proclaiming that many of the ingredients banned in the EU, like rocket fuel, are never used in beauty products. (This was the exact same talking point used five years prior in a hearing on Capitol Hill by the beauty industry trade association when defending our "strong" 1938 law.)

I pointed out that some of the EU's banned ingredients, like certain parabens, phthalates, and hydroquinone, were widely used in the United States, including in beauty products. And just because rocket fuel was listed as a banned substance (for reasons I didn't know either) didn't mean the whole point was moot. My takeaway: Europeans were provided stronger, even if imperfect, protections by their governments compared to the United States. Meanwhile, the cosmetic chemist's "fact-checker" was actively working the chat among the panelists, providing links to support whatever the cosmetic chemist was saying.

She had a staffed operation. My tank was empty.

I quickly changed my tact as I read the room. Because the virtual audience was being so whipped up by the cosmetic chemist (the comments section was a steady stream of praise for her forceful and smug retorts), I tried to sound more measured so I didn't come off as the irrational extremist among the panelists. This "pick your battles" strategy had served me well as a lobbyist and organizer, but here it was falling flat—the extremes were just too loud.

About halfway through the "debate," I shut down. Like, completely shut down. I didn't try to jump in and respond to the misinformation being shared, and I didn't swoop in to save the junior marketing person who was clumsily trying to defend the clean market. For years I had relished and crushed these types of moments, but now I had gone dead inside. It felt like sweeping sand at the beach. On this day, tired from debating the same things for over fifteen years, I realized that the mushrooming of misinformation in a digital world was something I could never tackle alone.

It was the wrong time to fail, and the wrong audience to fail with. My poor showing helped make the case to these journalists that "clean beauty is in fact BS." Only in the last five minutes of the hour-long panel did I muster the strength to shut down the most vocal panelist, though it was too little too late.

She had ended her closing argument by stating that it was unethical to imply that ingredients in beauty products weren't safe. The line about "ethics" hit me in my core.

Moving past my postpartum, sleep-deprived fog, I closed by saying, with force and attitude, "I think it's unethical to turn a blind eye and say that anything that questions the status quo is all 'fearmongering.' To say everything is safe for everyone when we have clear, peer-reviewed evidence showing there are disproportionate impacts to vulnerable populations such as pregnant women, children, and people of color, *that's* unethical." I ended with a warning about social media, saying it was also unethical to distill this debate down into black-and-white, fifteen-second social media posts, when the science is anything but simple."

The fire that normally showed up for me in these moments appeared fleetingly. But I closed the Zoom call disappointed and embarrassed. The panel experience solidified for me that we had entered a new and frightening era of the fight when influencers unwittingly (and wittingly) did the work of the chemical industry and everyone had their own "science" to reinforce their worldview.

Early in my career, when I was lobbying for consumer safety bills, the enemy was obvious. The chemical industry lobbyists were easy to spot and open about who they were and what they were defending. Now the enemy was everywhere and disguised as an influencer, making it nearly impossible for people to know what was true. The rules of the game had changed, and I wasn't sure how to combat this new Goliath.

What also depressed me was that those who should have been doing their due research diligence—journalists and editors—were falling down on their jobs. Many beauty editors and journalists had begun writing slanted articles and giving a large platform to cosmetic chemists and media-hungry dermatologists instead of quoting the scientists doing the actual research on how chemicals affect our health. As soon as the lead editor of one popular beauty outlet started hating on clean, the rest fell into line.

I discovered several months before the panel that some of the shift in press coverage was the direct result of seeds of doubt that had been planted by the mainstream beauty industry and its trade association. One afternoon, skimming through Instagram stories for my daily warp-speed tour of what my digital world was up to, I noticed that many of the beauty journalists I followed were attending a conference hosted by the beauty industry's trade association, the Personal Care Products Council (PCPC).

The PCPC had invited these professionals to its annual educational conference to promote understanding of the "real science" promulgated by social media and old-school toxicologists. While much more moderate and tame than the chemical industry's trade association (the ACC), the PCPC was funded by large older beauty brands that were mostly interested in maintaining the status quo. I had a bad feeling as I studied the editors' posts. One person showed a video of the registration table and the name tags of the people attending. My stomach dropped—the dozens of faces and names of editors that flashed before me were all people I knew, people with

whom I'd spent a considerable amount of time over the years educating them on the dirty details, people whose writing I respected.

Over the next few days I carefully monitored these journalists'
social content, which clued me in to the information they were being presented with. The PCPC had set up several panels for the press
to attend, and among the topics covered was the uniform safety
of ingredients in beauty products. Their panels were filled with
toxicologists from credible universities and dermatologists (most
of whom had their own beauty lines). Not a single environmental
health expert. Not a single panel on the well-researched risks of carcinogens, hormone disruptors, and mutagens in beauty products.
My heart sank.

I had the rude awakening that the press would now require
as much attention and ongoing education as elected officials. The
swell of progress fueled by one of the most important pillars of
movement—the press—had started to ebb. Many of the editors
and writers and press outlets I counted on to be good stewards of
the science were turning into dismissers themselves. They'd not
always gotten it right before—again, the science is complicated and
nuanced—but this was an entire sector swallowing whole lies and
regurgitating them for their followers.

It's diabolically brilliant in a way: the chemical industry hasn't
needed to budget nearly as much for PR efforts recently as in years
past since a fleet of "sci comms" and beauty editors and influencers
are now doing that job for them.

To the average person, the shift in press coverage was subtle,
perhaps undetectable, and even in circles where it should have been
noted, not many people seemed to be paying attention. Scientists
were doing what they should, conducting peer-reviewed research on
the health effects of chemicals. My old colleagues in the nonprofit
community were so underfunded and focused on the traditional

enemy (trade associations and the politicians in their pockets) that they weren't tracking the shift in narrative in beauty publications and social media feeds.

For me, it was like seeing a train wreck and turning to my allies, only to find them all looking the other way.

To be clear, I was not unaware that some of the media had been biased for quite some time. But an independent press using facts as their true north was indispensable to getting this complicated issue properly communicated to the masses. The founders of this country clearly outlined that an independent press is also critical to an educated electorate, which is foundational for a healthy democracy.

I took some solace in the fact that there were still highly skilled investigative journalists exposing certain truths to the public in publications such as the *New York Times*, the *Atlantic*, and *ProPublica*. I also saw that the morning and evening news shows of major networks continued to broadcast recall alerts about high levels of toxic chemicals in certain products and in our drinking water and soil. Still, I felt burdened by the sense that there was something more I could be doing from my perch, considering the relationships I'd already developed with so many of these editors and writers.

Sitting in the backyard on Saturday, I called my chatty, Gucci-wearing PR maven, now a close friend, for some advice. Squinting from the sun, I watched my eldest daughter bounce on the trampoline while I explained that these editors were at the center of an alarming cultural tipping point, and I asked her, "Do you think any of these writers realize they are now pumping out talking points from the chemical industry?"

Her response was quick: "I think they have no idea. None of these writers want to report things incorrectly or be a mouthpiece for the chemical industry."

I'd come to appreciate her as a conversation partner, always ready to engage, and I found myself sharing my deepest fears with her, exploring scenarios that I'd been wary of considering but that now seemed more possible than ever before. "So much of the work we've done to protect public health and the environment is at risk of being rolled back, or the forward march could wane. Yes, we've had a long list of important state wins, and TSCA reform passed, but federal reform isn't done, and cosmetics reform is still hanging in the balance."

She had an idea, the kernel of something that would be key to re-energizing me and getting things back on track for Camp Pragmatist. "Lindsay, let's do what we always have—hit this thing head on," she brainstormed. "If we are concerned that some of this press coverage is slanting in a way that will slow our progress, we should make sure all of these journalists have access to the right information, the right scientists, and the facts, which speak for themselves."

I felt that familiar spark get rekindled. She was right—we could turn this ship around with some targeted efforts. Over the next few weeks we pulled together a series of one-on-one phone calls with prominent journalists and editors covering toxic chemicals in beauty products, calls that had no agenda other than getting away from the black-and-white "clean beauty is BS" thinking and leaning into the gray areas and what we knew to be true according to strong science. This wasn't just my fight, nor was it Beautycounter's to tackle alone. We had to invest as much time with the press as we did with grassroots and elected officials to educate them.

On the calls, we opened up the floor for questions, unpacked them carefully, and offered to put writers and editors in touch directly with the Swans, Trasandes, and Zotas of the world for a deeper dive into the science. As in my conversations with swing voters, my goal wasn't to shame anyone publicly in a conference or panel (which is why I decided to forgo a group press event) or aggressively force facts down their throats, but to simply give them an opportunity to learn what years of dedicated research had revealed.

Over the next few months, the anti-clean coverage slowed down. We were breaking through.

I was intent on keeping the alignment strong between the press, the consumer market, the grassroots organizations, and the lobbyists because, with an understanding of the trajectory of passing federal legislation, I recognized the window of opportunity that was opening up for us. We'd been at exactly this precipice with TSCA—that moment when we'd made enough progress with a cross-section of industry players to have a really good shot at passing reform. Despite the backsliding in press coverage and the emergence of extreme influencers, we were getting close to pulling the trigger. Hill staff (the drivers of the bus) could soon look to all the major stakeholders and feel confident about calling the bill for a vote and hopefully making it law.

The signs were all there. Despite the political fractures and intolerances plaguing the country, the bipartisan grassroots base in support of federal beauty reform was still mostly intact and vocal. Hill offices were still working together in a bipartisan manner to find a compromise bill everyone could live with. The news cycle picked up again, having covered emerging issues like benzene (a carcinogen) in dry shampoo and the science showing that Black women who used certain hair dyes faced a 45 percent higher risk of breast cancer. The marketplace was also doing its thing: the exploding global clean beauty market was estimated to hit $7.2 billion in 2022.

Groups such as the Environmental Working Group, Beautycounter, the Personal Care Products Council (yes, they were at the negotiation table), and smaller trade associations (shout-out to the Handcrafted Soap & Cosmetic Guild, quite vocal as it turned out) were all weighing in on what their ideal version of reform looked like. It was the strongest signal yet that we were close, because for any major reform to happen a wide swath of stakeholders must sit down with each other and work out the policy differences before getting to any version of a final bill.

Last but not least, the fatigue factor was setting in—in this case, helpfully so—to play its pivotal role. Hill staff from both parties had been meeting for years to hash out compromise language to update our 1938 laws, and they were flagging. As odd as it sounds, this too gave me hope, because it meant that the cost of sunken returns was kicking in—things were becoming "do or die." It was now or never.

Fueling the urgency was the ticking of the congressional clock. It was late 2022, and if they didn't agree on a final bill package soon, the bill would have to be reintroduced in 2023, and the process would have to start all over again. (Any bill introduced needs to be voted on within the two-year period of any given Congress; otherwise, it has to be reintroduced.) It was unthinkable that all that work should go to waste.

And it didn't.

On an evening in December 2022, when I was at my parents' house for the Christmas holiday, I glanced down at my phone to see an incoming text from a colleague: "I have final bill language, need your perspective." Seeing the words "final bill" instantly shook me out of my holiday food coma. With a belly full of sugar cookies and wine, I asked my husband to watch the kids and give me some time while I learned the final details of the bill package.

I walked into the bedroom where we were staying, suitcases open, the bed unmade, and moved the clothes strewn on the floor to clear a spot of carpet to plunk down and call my colleague. Pulling a pen out of my purse and a scrap of paper from the trash can, I wrote down the details of the compromise bill: it allowed the FDA to recall unsafe products (yes!); it required companies to actually have a safety rationale for their ingredients versus the rubber-stamping that had given a free pass to the majority of ingredient decisions to date (an imperfect but small step forward); it authorized a study on key ingredients like PFAS and talc in cosmetics (it was clear that we knew enough to ban them, but I'll never say no to more research); and it required ingredient transparency for products sold online and those used by salon professionals (a great start—it didn't nix the poison stuff, but it at least gave us a heads-up about what was in there).

What wasn't included in the bill (and reader, this is where we are now, a big reason why I wrote this book): explicitly enabling the FDA to assess ingredients for safety (though it preserved states' ability to continue to pass their own bans); explicitly banning the worst chemicals, especially those targeted at women of color; and requiring companies to fully disclose their fragrance blends (so consumers would no longer be in the dark about whether or not there were toxic chemicals in those formulas).

As I looked at the notes I scribbled down, my colleague asked, "Do you think this is enough?"

Suddenly I was in Andy's position several years back on TSCA reform. A nine-year investment in the policy change had come down to an hour-long phone call in which I, as a stakeholder and someone with a 10,000-foot view, was being asked if there would be support for a bill that didn't fix all of the problems with toxic chemicals in beauty products.

Thinking through the merits of the policy that was read out loud to me, the many wins for public health included, and the clock that was running out for Congress to act, I delivered my verdict. "It would be a big step forward." I gave the policy my blessing.

Looking out the window, I watched as snow softly fell on the pine trees. The laughter from my family was muffled on the other side of the door, and holiday music was playing. Taking a moment for the news to sink in, I thought back to the early days when I arrived at Beautycounter's office in crumpled clothes and with a broken heart, not sure if I'd made the right decision in going over to the corporate side. I rewound images of the small groups of people we would turn out for events, groups that grew in size over time. I pictured Gregg testifying before the House of Representatives in a patriotic red dress. Feeling that familiar sense of pride for our collective hard work and, as a card-carrying pragmatist, a twinge from knowing our work is never really done, my mind shifted to the calls I needed to make to key people who deserved a heads-up that a final bill would soon be crossing the finish line. Many thanks were in order; this work is always a team effort.

My heart raced as I called Gregg first to break the news. I told her the deal was about to be final and walked her through the details. It was the best holiday gift we could have received, as well as fitting that a moment this big would happen when the majority of the world was spending time with their family. That was, after all, what fueled this work—the desire and the right to live healthy lives so we could spend meaningful time with the ones we love most.

"Gregg, this whole journey with Beautycounter has been far from easy, but we helped pass the first major reform to make beauty products safer in over eighty years."

She was silent for a short moment, an eternity given her fast-talking nature, and then she said, "I've never been good about celebrating the wins, I'm always on to the next thing. But I'm going to take in this moment. We did it, Lindsay."*

On December 23, 2022, a final bill to update the FDCA passed, nine years after Representative Schakowsky first introduced her bill and just one year less than the ten years I had told Gregg it would take. The legislation, called MoCRA (the Modernization of Cosmetics Reform Act—bills often take on new names as the legislative process unfolds), was a huge victory, the most significant expansion of the FDA authority to regulate cosmetics since 1938, a feat that many thought was impossible in a partisan Congress that shies away (and still does) from giving government agencies more power.

MoCRA's passage showed me that we still have a voice in our democracy, that grassroots organizing, consumer influence, and committed politicians of all stripes can move the needle. It reminded me that old-fashioned dealmaking—opposing entities like public health groups and trade associations and old and new businesses all compromising in order to take a step forward—is still possible. The dominoes were starting to fall in the right direction.

In a sign of sustained progress in 2023, the FDA announced it was taking steps to chip away at the list of issues not immediately solved by MoCRA, including a proposed ban on formaldehyde in hair-straightening treatments.

On days when I want to pat us all on the back and throw in the towel, I'm reminded that the most exposed and vulnerable communities, those who can't shop around the problem, are still in the firing line. The kids I saw playing on the polluted playground in Galveston. Vi's community struggling to keep their way of life alive without exposing themselves to unprecedented levels of toxic chemicals. Chemical companies are still operating at full tilt, concocting

---

* Gregg Renfrew is currently the founder and CEO of Counter Beauty.

"regrettable replacements" to swap out when only one specific toxic chemical gets banned instead of an entire class.

Unsexy product categories, like carpeting, are still polluting our homes by the pound. (While most flame retardants are no longer used in couches, recycled polyurethane foam is used for the majority of carpet padding, recirculating this persistent class of chemicals in our homes.) And there are still no widely accepted methods that cosmetic companies can use to accurately test for relevant PFAS and other emerging contaminants in makeup.

For all the progress we've made, including TSCA and MoCRA, our work is far from done. But don't worry—as uphill a battle as it seems, I know how to get us there.

10

YOU

IN THE SUMMER OF 2018—A COUPLE OF YEARS AFTER TSCA passed—I found myself driving a small jerky rental car through the streets of Newark, nauseous and pregnant with my first child, on my way to doing an impossible task: delivering a eulogy for one of my closest friends and mentors, and our movement's leader, Andy Igrejas. After a hard one-and-a-half-year battle with brain cancer, Andy lost his life. His wife, Susan, asked me to deliver a eulogy, with a focus on speaking to the accomplishments of his career.

Parking on the street, the row houses lined up close to the sidewalk, I noticed a few small markets and Italian diners flanking the street. I entered the funeral salon, a home repurposed as a space to honor those who had passed. Dark browns and maroons dominated the space. The whole setting resembled a scene from *The Sopranos*.

Everyone took their seats, and shakily, I walked up to the podium and turned to face Andy's close friends and family. Within the first few sentences, my lips started to quiver. I avoided looking at my former colleagues in the audience, knowing I would break down in tears if our eyes locked. I shared how Andy was the silent hero who put consumer safety issues on the map. I walked through the early days of his career discussing the environmental laws he helped pass in New Jersey and California, and how he led our coalition of advocates to one of the largest national environmental and health victories of the decade, overhauling TSCA. I wanted to make sure that his legacy was crystal clear to everyone there: Andy's relentless commitment to public health and safety was a gift to humanity.

Afterward, his extended family and friends from high school approached me, and they all said the same thing: they had no idea that Andy had done this monumental work. To them, he was just a guy from New Jersey who liked cooking Portuguese fried cod fritters and making his friends laugh through animated storytelling and impersonations.

The truth is that Andy was just like a lot of us: a person who cared about a cause and decided to do something about it. While Andy made a career out of removing toxic chemicals from our products, communities, air, and water, his work and success were possible only because he galvanized individuals like you and me to participate in that work. As Representative Schakowsky says, and as I've learned from decades doing this work too, nothing passes—nothing improves—without enough of us demanding change.

I'm often asked how I find hope in a career filled with depressing realities. The honest truth is that I have become more hopeful as I've pressed on. I have consistently seen the power of the marketplace and consumer behavior, and how the voices of people have won out over the deep pockets of corporate donors. I've witnessed our ability to rise above the toxic extremist voices hammering each other on social media. Let me walk you through the hope and empowerment I see in all of those areas—the market, our laws, our culture. I want you to feed off these facts and wins as fuel for the collective actions, small but mighty, that I list in the resources section. These actions build on the legacy that Andy left us and that every scientist, public servant, and activist I've highlighted in this book has contributed to. It's our turn.

The Market

Your purchasing choices have profound impact in two major ways. First, your spending power convinces companies to create clean products. We saw the clean beauty market go from nothing in the early 2010s to a $10 billion-plus global market in less than fifteen years. That was due to consumer pressure and power. When you prioritize a safer version of a brand's product line over the less-safe version, companies start to look at other offerings through the clean lens. As crass as it sounds, if clean is profitable, companies will follow the money. I can also tell you, as someone who's worked on the inside of companies, that they listen when you give feedback on their ingredients, packaging and sourcing practices. This is exactly what happened with the toy, household cleaner, beauty, and now supplement markets. Your dollars—and your reasons for making these purchases—matter.

Second, and equally important: bringing safer products into your home has a quantifiable impact on your health. Research shows that reducing your exposure to certain toxic chemicals with short half-lives reduces the levels in your body—in some cases quite quickly. The Silent Spring Institute and Breast Cancer Prevention

Partners looked at the impacts of removing all food packaging from families' lives for three days. The results, which were peer-reviewed and published, showed a 66 percent reduction in bisphenol A. (The reverse is true too: as soon as these families resumed their normal diets, their levels of BPA rose again.)

We see the same steep drop when people swap in cleaner personal care products. A study from the University of California at Berkeley followed Latina teenagers who replaced conventional beauty and personal care products—those containing parabens and oxybenzone—with clean versions for three days. Astoundingly, their levels of parabens plummeted by 44 percent, and their oxybenzone levels dropped by 36 percent.

These findings should give you confidence that you're not flushing your money down the drain when you shop for safer products.

I haven't spent much time discussing pesticides in this book, but for the dismissers out there pushing back on eating organic food (yes, they are also doing that), you should know that plenty of research has linked exposures to certain pesticides like organophosphates to harmful impacts on children's brains and motor development. Little, lighter bodies (including those developing in utero) bear a heavier burden, and immature organs may not be able to remove pesticides and other toxic chemicals as well as adult organs. (Note that the USDA organic certification doesn't ban all pesticides, just the most toxic ones.)

Eating organic is not only about our health; it is just as much about protecting farmworkers, who face higher rates of cancer, infertility, and neurological disorders, all linked to pesticides. Farmworkers are often migrant workers from historically marginalized communities whose homes, schools, and ecosystems are also negatively impacted by pesticides. It's a double dose of poison.

Our Laws

I've made a strong case for the need for laws that hold polluters accountable, not only to protect people who buy and use their products but to safeguard the resources we all share—the air and water and soil. For a country built on a culture of individualism, thinking about and caring for the collective whole is sometimes hard. This is one of the underlying reasons the United States has trouble passing laws or taking actions that are in the best interest of the general public's health and not only of our own families. I get it—I'm mama bear too—but we are all connected. And the funny thing about toxic chemicals that find their way into the environment? They don't stop at state lines or stay inside certain zip codes.

If you're still wondering if laws have actually resulted in public health wins, if they really make that big of a difference, the answer is: absolutely. Let's look at the scientific proof:

When the United States banned lead from paint in 1978, the average blood level of lead in the US population dropped by 78 percent from 1978 to 1991. A study published in 2022 found that lead levels have continued to decline, falling from an average of 0.16 parts per million in the late '60s (when lead in gasoline was in peak use) to below 0.01 parts per million in 2021, in great part because the EPA mandated the removal of lead in gasoline beginning in 1975.

Another example comes from Dr. Zota—you met her in chapter 8—who published a peer-reviewed study looking at the urine levels of phthalates in the US population after the 2008 federal ban on certain phthalates in children's toys. (Thanks again, Representative Schakowsky!) Zota and her colleagues found that levels of the three phthalates banned (BBzP, DnBP, and DEHP) plummeted by an average of 20 to 40 percent over a span of eight years. Even though the ban covered only toys, the declines were found across the whole US population, not just in children, because companies saw the writing on the wall: when phthalates were banned in children's products, they started removing them across other product categories too. Interestingly, the three phthalates that were flagged in the law for further scientific review, along with a few others (DiBP, DnOP, DiDP and DiNP), all increased in the US population. Levels of DiNP rose a shocking 150 percent. This certainly suggests that companies switched from the banned phthalates to replacement chemicals that were not outright banned.

Our Culture

Culture is the factor that keeps me up at night because it is the most powerful and the least predictable. The ability of cultural movements to shape our world is immense, for better and for worse. I see glimmers of how our culture can push the clean movement for the better, but now—real talk—it's shifted in the other direction. Cultural trends like the latest workout class (barre class, anyone?) or music (when did yacht rock become so cool?) are relatively harmless. The problem comes in when groups of people become entrenched in a fixed worldview, unwilling to compromise even when faced with evidence to the contrary. Critical thinking goes out the window. Facts lose out to unyielding beliefs. Science gets dismissed. Empathy becomes muted.

I'm describing a person who is an idealogue, someone who always wants to see things their way and receives only information that confirms their values and politics. What does this have to do with the clean living movement? As you probably guessed, a lot.

The folks on the outer edges—the dismissers and perfectionists—have unintentionally become idealogues. For them, there is no longer nuance, no "hmmm, let me consider that differently," no "I didn't know that, so let me dig deeper." Idealogues want clear-cut battle cries and obvious stances that are easy to boil down to a meme, a bumper sticker, or a post.

Oversimplifying by making broad declarative statements doesn't fix the problem—it just fixes how you feel about it. The more people bring black-and-white thinking to matters of clean living, the harder it is to come together and focus, despite our differences, on the facts and fix what's broken. As I wrote in chapter 9, idealogues are alive and kicking on social media, where 140-character tweets and short-form Tik-Toks give all-or-nothing thinking a megaphone. Besides stoking divisions in our social feeds, idealogues also populate DC legislative chambers, causing gridlock. The disheartening reality: we are more divided than ever and triggered by everything, so much so that it's becoming harder and harder to enjoy a beer around the campfire with our politically diverse families.

Here's what keeps me in the ring, despite this dumpster fire we're in: research from the University of Pennsylvania's Damon Centola finds that the tipping point for social change happens when just 25 percent of a population embraces an idea. Obviously an idea can catch fire for better and for worse (fascism, anyone?), but reaching 25 percent is a doable benchmark.

And I know we can get there, because it's been done before. I was in college when I first learned how harmful ideological thinking can be and how to counter it. A professor introduced our class to Václav Havel, a dissident, writer, and movement builder in Czechoslovakia (now the Czech Republic) during the Soviet reign. Havel spoke out in both open and underground publications about how ideological thinking was contributing to the oppression of the Czech people and allowing the totalitarian regime to thrive. In recounting the conversations he had on the streets with people from wildly different backgrounds, he showed that it was not only possible but essential to listen to each other, to meet your audience where they were, and in doing so, an open and productive exchange of ideas. Using the power of ideas and words, Havel did what many considered impossible: he led the first peaceful throwdown of the Soviet government in 1989 by speaking to diverse audiences and holding up a mirror to the Czech people who had fallen prey to ideological thinking.

My hope is that we will hold up a mirror to our own behavior and its impact on our progress on environmental health issues. I can already hear you telling yourself that you do think critically, that this section isn't for you. The fact is that everyone has an inner idealogue who holds firm to some belief in a way that can end up hurting them or hurting society. When I look in my own mirror, I see I am not immune from ideological thinking.

So here's where I'd like to challenge you on the cultural front, and where I believe our greatest hope lies: question your deeply held beliefs through a critical lens. I want everyone, even the most righteous of readers, to do a gut check. Ask yourself, "How am I receiving information? Am I part of the problem?" Before you post on social media, ask yourself if it's that simple. When you're reading a post—even from your favorite content creator—think critically. I'm not suggesting you become judgmental, but rather more discerning. Strive for meaningful dialogues with people you don't agree with.

Our health hangs in the balance as we decide whether or not we can rise above our own biases and assumptions. It's challenging but critical work because nothing is more valuable than our health. With a healthy body and mind, we can enjoy community, friendships, and the people we love. There's nothing more important than that.

Maybe you're a crunchy mama who is willing to consider that an anti-government mindset is one reason we're in this mess in the first place, and that perhaps there is a place for commonsense regulations that protect our bodies and our babies' bodies from toxic chemicals. You hold an incredible amount of power that you can use to hold your political party accountable (especially today) and show party leaders that their base does care about commonsense regulations on toxic chemicals.

Ever since the vaccine debates, many have embraced the battle cry that you should challenge everything and "do your research." This approach is tricky, for it seems to embrace the idea of being a critical thinker. But depending on where that "research" is coming from—one-off studies from an esoteric journal, industry-funded studies, influencers or even politicians who are twisting the facts—it can still feed ideological thinking and become a form of confirmation bias. Ask yourself: Am I searching for facts? Or am I uninterested in whether the info is credible or not and merely searching for a position that reinforces my own views?

Maybe you're a perfectionist who, after considering your own biases and assumptions, can now take a step back and see that it's not just about filling your home with safer products to protect your family, but that critical social justice issues are at play and we need broader action. Maybe you can roll up your sleeves and, instead of just placing orders for new products, also start placing calls to your elected officials, to ask for strong state and federal oversight of toxic chemicals.

Maybe you're a dismisser who can resolve to brush up on the scientific consensus around exposures to certain toxic chemicals and approach content about consumer safety with more nuance.

You may then realize that it's not all fearmongering. And that dismissing the issue outright actively ignores threats to the health of those who live in fenceline communities near the production of chemicals.

Maybe you're none of the above. Perhaps you're just an overwhelmed parent or student who is on board with a lot of what I've shared but not sure where to begin or whether you can make a difference with the five minutes you have to spare. You can. I've met so many different types of people in my twenty-plus years in the trenches who have made small, incremental shifts in their thinking and behaviors, away from the extremes and toward the center. We have much to feel good about and celebrate so far.

Okay, buckle up. While all of the signs of progress fill me with hope (and hopefully you too), we're only halfway done with our fight. I want to leave you with an eyes-wide-open assessment of where the environmental health movement stands and what lies ahead in the second half of our mission.

We are at a dangerous precipice where we are at risk of having the chemical and consumer safety laws people fought so hard for watered down or reversed altogether. To put it bluntly, the science on how chemicals in products affect our health is being dismissed, ignored, or actively contorted as I type this. We've seen the US Supreme Court and the Trump administration make decisions that rolled back significant protections for the environment and our health, laws that took generations of effort to enact. (I can feel some readers bristling— this is a statement of fact, not partisan commentary.) How well TSCA and MoCRA are implemented and enforced by the EPA and FDA is largely dependent on who is appointed to those agencies. The EPA's chemical safety program is currently run by ACC veteran Nancy Beck. Within the first two months of Trump's second term, rollbacks were actioned removing progress on PFAS and lead in pipes. As I was finalizing this chapter, executive orders were signed to roll back programs and protections for environmental justice communities, some of whom you met in the pages of this book. After decades of work to enact these laws, the protections they provide are at real risk of being watered down or eliminated entirely.

Scientists are retreating from the public eye for fear of being maligned. Funding for nonprofits working on the front lines has slowed. Information fatigue is causing people to give up and tune out. Safety and science have become politicized, and many people can no longer find ways to discuss these problems with family members and friends who have different political or lifestyle views than their own.

Many companies that once positioned themselves as clean have removed the mention of it from their brand descriptions and social media handles for fear of turning off customers. Sadly, clean has become a dirty word in some circles. The backlash coming from the dismissers is working. Many more brands are claiming to be "nontoxic" and "natural" and "dermatologist tested" but doing the bare minimum instead of learning what it takes to formulate safe and clean products. This isn't just about making federal standards for how brands can use these marketing terms (though that would be nice), but a whole supply chain overhaul. And the reality is that some of the strongest laws have come from actions by state governments.

The soaps and makeup and cookware we buy when we stock up at big-box stores, while safer than they were twenty years ago, still require that we be scientists in order to ID the least toxic options.

Even when specific toxic chemicals are banned, regrettable substitutions often appear instead.

Some of the most toxic classes of chemicals, like PFAS, are still legally allowed, and they have become global pollutants that make it hard for clean companies to devise formulas free of problematic contaminants. People in vulnerable communities continue to get poisoned by the factories making the very chemicals and plastics we bring into our homes. And as long as there remains no required ingredient transparency for product categories like fragrances, furniture, fashion, building materials, children's toys, and baby cribs, we are all left in the dark.

I don't care what political affiliation you call home—this is happening to all of us.

Here is my ask, the reason I wrote this book and stole time away from my family and friends to sound the alarm. Now is a critical moment for individuals to get engaged, or re-engaged, in this fight. People who have been involved in this movement for decades need your help so that we can stop poisoning ourselves and future generations.

We must remove the burden of asking people to be their own federal agencies and put the onus where it belongs: on our government and companies to do better. The resources section at the end of this book provides a playbook for how to do just that. I've made the guidelines simple and effective, and you can tailor them to your level of interest and availability—a choose-your-own-adventure activism. You don't have to engage in it all day every day or spend a lot of money or do a TED talk or make a career out of it (unless you really want to, in which case DM me). You only need to care enough to do something.

Leaving Andy's memorial, I went to my rental car and sat and cried. (I am not a public crier—I hate having to assure people that I'm okay.) I knew this day was coming, but I still couldn't believe that we were all breathing air and Andy was not. I smiled, knowing he would have made a joke right about now about the polluted air in Newark. (He wouldn't have been wrong—living in a hub for transit activity and trash incineration, Newark's kids have double the national rate of asthma. The city is working on it.)

I'd always felt a responsibility to safeguard the planet and its people—heck, I'd made a career out of it—but now, in an Andy-less world, I experienced a deepening sense of obligation. There weren't a lot of people I knew with the resilience and drive for world betterment that Andy brought to the work, day in and day out. Would our movement suffer? I felt the baby kick and resolved that it would not. Andy spent his time on this planet trying to leave it in a better state than when he arrived. I would do the same for my daughters, and I hoped they would eventually do the same for their own children. The torch gets passed, and it's up to us to decide how far we are going to run with it before our chance to light the way burns out.

Losing a close friend, a child, a cousin, sibling, or parent is incredibly painful. And the desire for more time with them is usually the one thing we all want when we reflect on the life lost. That's really what this work is about. Protecting our collective public health so that we can all have a little more time with the people we love.

I fight so I can have more moments like the fleeting minute of peace when my daughter floats on her back in the bath, staring at the ceiling, quietly swishing her hair back and forth. So that I don't need to think twice about the workers and communities impacted by the chemicals used to treat my rain jacket. So that I don't worry about chemical exposures when I watch my kids squeal and bounce on a vinyl inner tube being dragged behind a boat at the family cabin.

Fueling my tank for the second half of this fight is knowing this movement, given its tremendous breadth, is filled with thousands of Andy Igrejases, Arlene Blums, Shanna Swans, Robert Bilotts, Pam Millers, Vi Waghiyis, Juan Parrases, Gregg Renfrews, and Jan Schakowskys.

Perhaps most importantly, the movement contains millions of people like you.

TAKE ACTION

WHEREVER YOU ARE ON THIS JOURNEY, IT'S THE PER-fect starting point. Remember, I started as a skeptic, so you don't have to get into full-on activist mode right away (though I would love that). Because none of these suggestions provide the full solution on their own, I encourage you to pick something from each area to commit to doing regularly. We are all worth the effort.

Safer Ways to Shop the Market

Many people are not in a position to shop their way to safety, and as a matter of social justice, we should aim to fix this problem for everyone, not just the wealthy. That said, there are ways anyone can shop the market for safer products:

Buy half of what you typically consume. This is the best and highest-impact way you can help reduce the demand for and use of toxic chemicals. It's also the simplest. We (including myself) buy too much shit, and every product has impacts on human and planetary health. With the commodification of wellness and health, even of sustainability, we all need to re-assess our consumption instead of buying into (literally) the idea that we need every product the market introduces to us.

Buy secondhand. Repair products (like we used to). Maybe skip an iPhone model or two or three before you purchase your next one. And before you pop that next item into your cart, ask yourself: Do I need this? If not, who might be impacted if I click "purchase"?

Shop some of my favorite brands. This is a quickly moving landscape, so you can find my brand and product recommendations online at heyhilde.com.

Look for specific certifications. These certifications—while imperfect—are the strongest for assessing ingredient safety and contaminants: EWG VERIFIED for beauty and personal care products (there is also an app version); MADE SAFE for other product categories like children's toys and cleaners; EPA Safer Choice for cleaners and other household products; Clean Label Project, which tests supplements and protein powder for over two hundred common contaminants; Cradle to Cradle Certified Gold Material Health (for furniture and building materials); and GreenScreen Certified (for various product categories)

Shop at retailers leading the way. The Mind the Store campaign, which, thanks to the team at Toxic Free Future, is still going strong (your legacy lives on, Andy). Mind the Store ranks retailers annually based on the strength of their policies to remove toxic chemicals from their shelves. Although a top ranking doesn't ensure that all of a retailer's products are clean, you're voting with your dollar to support those retailers who are stepping up and taking this issue seriously. Visit retailerreportcard.org.

Prioritize. Perfection and total control are illusions. Focus on products that are larger sources of exposure to the most toxic chemicals, items such as couches, mattresses, and cookware. If your budget can cover only some clean beauty products, prioritize the ones that stay on your skin all day (lotion, makeup) and worry less about those that rinse off, such as shampoo and conditioner. And know that safer does not always mean expensive; good old-fashioned white distilled vinegar (acidic, antimicrobial) is an effective way to clean your countertops, floors, and toilets.

Be wary of consumer apps. Clearya and EWG Skin Deep are the two strongest, science-based apps that assess product and chemical safety. Some others, like Yuka, Think Dirty, and Good Guide, are well intentioned but fail to give you complete and accurate safety ratings. Although most of the consumer apps that cover a variety of product categories (with a heavy emphasis on beauty) were developed by individuals aiming to offer real guidance, their developers have limited, if any, experience in the science of environmental health, product formulation, or accurate assessment of risk. Most don't consider how much an ingredient is used within and across the formulas or its intended use on the body. As we know, all of this matters, since the science is complicated and nuanced. For those apps applying scientific research results to a product ranking, it's easy to miss the mark, especially as most are not staffed with environmental health scientists. Nearly all of the apps on the market are not reflective of the science and can undermine those brands doing the real work.

I'll give you an example: the Yuka and Think Dirty apps give a "poor" ranking to any product that includes the preservative phenoxyethanol. Most personal care products need a preservative to prevent the growth of mold, yeast, and bacteria. That is a matter of safety. However, the vast majority of chemical preservatives rank high on the hazard scale because they need to kill these unwanted microbes. So responsible brands must perform a balancing act—choosing safer preservatives (phenoxyethanol being one of them) to protect the integrity of the formula while also protecting your health. (EU regulations show that phenoxyethanol can be safely used at concentrations under 1 percent, which is how most brands use it.) But a few misguided studies about phenoxyethanol that were neither conducted scientifically nor applicable to its use in beauty products have stirred up the internet and led Yuka and Think Dirty to inappropriately ding products that contain the chemical.

View consumer product testing with a discerning eye. Headlines frequently hit social media when consumer products are tested for various toxic chemicals. Having conducted third-party testing myself as an activist and inside various companies, I can report that testing methods, equipment, results, and how they are presented to the world greatly matter. Some outlets are more trustworthy than others, including Consumer Reports and the Good Housekeeping Institute. And research published in peer-reviewed scientific literature, though not especially accessible for lay readers, is typically transparent about testing methods and potential limitations and has had scientific advisers review the process. Bloggers and influencers, however, deserve a closer look.

A few things to consider: Brands should be actively testing their own products for relevant chemicals and contaminants, which is not happening enough. Consumers also need to know that contaminants, even for clean brands, are impossible to avoid altogether. Certain PFAS, heavy metals, pesticides, phthalates, formaldehyde, and parabens can easily show up at contaminant levels in, yes, even clean products.

Since there's a perverse disincentive for brands not to test—ignorance is bliss—the brands that do test should be supported in this effort to put their customers first, not outed with "gotcha" takedowns. (Can you tell I've witnessed leading clean brands doing the real work unfairly targeted, and been irritated by it?) Take testing from non-scientist-run websites with a grain of salt. And continue to ask your elected officials for more regulation of upstream supply chain partners, which helps solve the issue of contaminants that are hard for even the best brands to entirely control. I know it's not sexy, but it always comes back to policy.

Know the basics for key product categories. While there is a lot of nuance to this topic, tried-and-true, high-level consumer tips to keep in mind while shopping are on page 229.

Suss Out the Greenwashers

If a brand says its products are "clean" or "sustainable" or uses related marketing language, see if it defines these terms. One of the best confirmations that a brand is legit is the presence of a dedicated page on its site that defines terms like "clean," "sustainable," etc., in detail. Any clean standard should go beyond retailer certifications and include explicit language about how they screen ingredients for safety—a precautionary approach is the North Star—as well as details about testing programs (many "clean" brands are not actively screening their own ingredients or testing for things like heavy metals). If the brand sets public goals (such as reducing plastic or working toward climate goals around carbon reduction), it should also have details on how it's going to hit those goals and transparently track progress. Anything short of sharing these important details is greenwashing.

Check LinkedIn to see if a brand has hired any safety or sustainability experts. You would be surprised how many brands are built on a sustainable and clean platform and yet haven't hired anyone with senority or the expertise to make sure real work on this front is happening. The lack of a dedicated staff is the biggest red flag, indicating that the brand thinks of the clean/green category only as a marketing exercise.

Push Brands Toward Safer and More Sustainable Products

Ask brands to participate in the Chemical Footprint Project. The Chemical Footprint Project is the only comprehensive third-party assessment of a company's chemical safety program that is robust and inclusive of all the complexities covered in this book. Major brands have participated, including Walmart, HP, Beautycounter, Target, and HermanMiller. The power of the Chemical Footprint Project is that it is an objective assessment of a company's overall approach to safety and testing. In other words, if any of the faux clean companies went through this assessment, they would be given a long "to-do" list and large slices of humble pie. (Many greenwashers are not malicious. I often see CEOs and founders who think they are leading in safety and sustainability but just have no idea what is really required to make that a reality.)

The Chemical Footprint Project is not focused on scoring a finished product; instead, it thoroughly analyzes the strength of a company's overall approach to managing chemicals. Does it have a restricted substance list, and if so, how strong is it? What is its approach to testing and risk? How does it incorporate all of these steps into the product development process? Answers to questions like these provide a company with a thorough roadmap for doing better. Some brands, for transparency, have even shared their results publicly.

You can help increase transparency and shine a light on green-washers by asking brands to participate. View the brands with the best-rated chemical safety programs on Chemicalfootprint.org.

ASK YOUR FAVORITE COMPANIES THESE QUESTIONS:

* Can you share more details about your safety and testing program? Do you take a precautionary "better safe than sorry" approach to formulating products, or do you implement traditional toxicology practices?

* Do you ban high hazard ingredients, as outlined by tools like GreenScreen and ChemFORWARD? (GreenScreen and ChemFORWARD are scientifically rigorous tools and organizations that assess ingredients by hazard level for human health and environmental impact.)

* Do you publish or share any safety test results with customers?

* Do you have any senior-level scientists or sustainability experts on staff to guide your formulating decisions and to reduce the company's overall negative health and environmental impacts?

* Will you participate in the Chemical Footprint Project so that consumers can have a third-party assessment of the strength of your safety program?

* How much visibility and traceability does your supply chain provide you?

* Do you issue an annual impact report that shares and tracks your progress on safety and sustainability issues?

＊ Do you have plans to seek the following certifications: EWG VERIFIED, MADE SAFE, EPA Safer Choice, or Clean Label Project?

A friendly note that a company's responses to these questions may not be easy to understand or even be real answers. The point of asking them is to put pressure on the company to take a precautionary approach to managing chemicals in its products and supply chains. Just by asking the question you are making a difference.

Help Pass Laws That Fix the Problem

Email and call Congress about this issue. As someone who witnessed the power of the electorate, I know it makes a difference. Here are the highest-impact ways to communicate with Congress (and why):

Send a personal email via the contact form on the site for your US senators and House representative. These seemingly old-school contact forms directly route your email to the staff member who is leading consumer safety and health issues for your elected officials. There are so few people who take the time to drop a personal email (it doesn't have to be long) that these communications hold a lot of weight, and with the right people. The note can be as simple as this:

"I am a constituent and I learned about how toxic chemicals can be found in our consumer products, air, and water. I strongly urge you to stand up for and support legislation that would empower the EPA and FDA to protect consumers. Please take action to:

1. Ban the most toxic chemicals, such as PFAS, which are linked to widespread harm to human health and the environment.

2. Support efforts to close gaps in federal laws overseeing personal care and cosmetic safety, including those that close the fragrance loophole and hold the beauty industry supply chain accountable for harmful contaminants, and those that proactively address the harmful chemicals used in products targeted at people of color.

3. Establish health-protective limits on heavy metals and other contaminants in cosmetics and supplements.

4. Ensure that regulatory agencies responsible for protecting human health and the environment from harmful exposures are adequately resourced with funding and staff to do their job effectively.

I look forward to hearing back from you on this important issue."

Call Congress. As Representative Schakowsky shared, it takes only ten phone calls in a week to put an issue directly on the radar of your elected officials. By law, each call must be recorded and tallied. Not sure how to find your elected officials' phone numbers? Call the Capitol switchboard to be directly connected: (202) 224-3121. Your message can be as simple as this:

"Hi, I'm a constituent and I recently learned about toxic chemicals in our consumer products. I'm calling to ask that my representative support legislation to ban toxic chemicals from products, like the Safer Beauty Bill package introduced

by Representative Schakowsky. Can you please share my feed-
back directly?"

Sign online petitions and emails, but hack the system. Many nonprofit
organizations send out emails asking you to email Congress, and
there is skepticism that the form emails actually work. The short
answer is that some Hill offices do block mass emails that have the
same formatting. Some do not. To make sure a form petition or
email breaks through, slightly change the contents of the email.
You will notice that most organizations let you read the email
and edit it before you hit send. Changing the first sentence can be
enough to make sure it gets to the right people.

**Vote, and learn about where the candidates stand on consumer safety
issues.** Before someone gets elected to office, or when they are seeking reelection, they take note of the issues they are asked about
on the campaign trail. You can email a candidate's campaign asking where they stand specifically on consumer safety and environmental health. Drop your question into the comment form on the
candidate's website. Something such as the following will let them
know you care about the issue and give you some intel:

> Dear Candidate X,
> I recently learned about the issue of toxic chemicals in everyday
> consumer products, and I want to know: Would you support state
> or federal regulations to protect our health from the hazardous
> toxic chemicals that are polluting our products and communities?

Write a letter to the editor. Elected officials monitor the opinion pages
of their local and state news publications as a way to stay in touch

with what their constituents care about. Feeling motivated? Head to the opinion page of your local newspaper and read the criteria for submitting a letter to the editor. State why you care about the issue—perhaps you read a recent report or you just welcomed your first baby—and include a clear ask of your elected officials. It can be as basic as, "It is my hope that our state and federal elected officials take the issue of toxic chemical pollution seriously and pass legislation to better protect public health so my kids can grow up in a safer world."

Run for office. A tall order, I know, but when I was interviewing Representative Schakowsky, she reminded me that women in particular (as backed by polling) consider themselves less qualified to run for office than their male counterparts. Clearly this isn't true, but it is part of the reason we have fewer elected officials who are women. If you're inspired to participate in a local PTA chapter or run for the school board, city council, or state government, go for it! The organization VoteRunLead.org is committed to helping first-time female candidates run . . . and win.

Find out if legislation is being proposed in your state to remove toxic chemicals from consumer products. Some of the strongest laws and best work on this topic is happening by leading public health and environmental nonprofits at the state level. You can find out how to get involved in your state by visiting: saferstates.org.

Follow and support the next steps in federal cosmetics safety legislation: Breast Cancer Prevention Partners (bcpp.org), Environmental Working Group (ewg.org), the Natural Resources Defense Council (nrdc.org), and WE ACT for Environmental Justice (weact.org).

Follow and support next steps to strengthen and uphold TSCA: For information, visit: Toxic-Free Future (toxicfreefuture.org), Environmental Defense Fund (edf.org), Earthjustice (earthjustice.org), and the NRDC (nrdc.org).

Challenge Your Own Black-and-White Thinking

The impacts of social media on our mental health have been well documented, but the role of carefully crafted algorithms in our lives runs much deeper. Polarizing content is prioritized, meaning algorithms are programmed not only to deliver posts similar to what you already like and share but to include content that is more extreme. And extreme content fuels more engagement.

Misinformation and disinformation go unchecked, and the echo chambers we have built for ourselves through the friends and people we follow—combined with the echo chambers being built for us by giant social media companies—have helped create the different realities we live in.

If you wonder how on earth your friend from high school could believe what she shares on social media, she is thinking the same of you. We've become polarized not only on the issues but in our feelings about the people whose position on those issues differs from ours, something social scientists call "affective polarization." Translation: "He is bad because he believes X, and I am good because I believe Y." When you're fed only content that affirms your beliefs, it's harder to find common ground and shared humanity.

Until social media companies develop protocols that diversify content and flag or ban misinformation, it's up to us to do that for ourselves.

Challenge your own ideology. I promise there is at least one belief you have gone all in on that could use some nuance. For starters, hold members of your own political party accountable. This may be hard, but it's an important step for all of us. Bucking ideological thinking requires constant vigilance and critical thinking. Just as there is no perfect person, there is no perfect party. Democrats, if you don't think your party is strong enough on workplace safety regulations or firearms in light of school shootings, call them. Republicans, if you're concerned that your party isn't supporting swift action on chemical safety or climate change, hold them accountable. Our founding fathers used the phrase "to form a more perfect union" in drafting the Constitution for a reason—constant improvement is a feature, not a glitch.

Prune your consumption. What apps can you delete? Do you really need three or can you make do with one? Which influencer accounts can you opt out of? (Hint: Do they promote black-and-white thinking? Unfollow.) Set boundaries for when you engage with social media content. Use a timer or a usage restriction app—yup, there's an app for that—or consider regular social media fasts. (Tip: delete apps from your phone so you can access them only from your web browser.)

Pause when you see political content you disagree with. When someone you respect posts something that produces a visceral reaction in you, give them a little grace before you jump to a conclusion or unfollow. Ask yourself if there is a reason they shared something that you may not fully understand. (Obviously, this doesn't apply to hate speech or dangerous conspiracy theories.) Remind yourself why you like this person regardless of their different political views.

Don't engage with problematic content. Doing so just lets more people see it. Resist falling into debates in comments sections. This is true not only for influencers and branded content but for friends and family.

Restrict teens' access to social media until they're sixteen. This recommendation comes from social psychologist Jonathan Haidt in his book *The Anxious Generation*. Restricting access at a young age can also reduce the political polarization of our youth by limiting their access to political content. Instead, encourage them to read the news from the sources listed below.

Donate and Support Organizations

The power of the individual cannot be underestimated, but we are so much stronger when we are mobilized around a shared call to action. The organizations featured in this book and below need your support, your resources (donate if you're able), your time (volunteer, show up to hearings), and your voice (tell your friends). They are also great sources for staying on top of the latest science and news.

THESE ARE SOME OF THE LEADING ORGANIZATIONS IN NEED OF YOUR SUPPORT:

Agents of Change*

Alaska Community Action on Toxics*

Asbestos Disease Awareness Organization

Black Women for Wellness*

Breast Cancer Prevention Partners*

California Healthy Nail Salon Collaborative

Center for Environmental Health

Center for Health, Environment & Justice

Center for International Environmental Law

Clean Water Action

Coming Clean

Earthjustice

Ecology Center

Environmental Defense Fund

Environmental Working Group

Green Science Policy Institute*

Indigenous Environmental Network

League of Conservation Voters

Louisiana Bucket Brigade

Natural Resources Defense Council*

Plastic Pollution Coalition

Silent Spring Institute*

Toxic-Free Future*

Texas Environmental Justice Advocacy Services*

WE ACT for Environmental Justice*

Women's Voices for the Earth

*Donations were made to these organizations as part of publishing this book, as they were featured and are home organizations for many of the experts interviewed.

Stay Informed

The body of environmental health research continues to grow, and sharing information is a key part of a growing social movement. As we have seen, when well-intended individuals spread misinformation, it can do a disservice to the larger movement and give the dismissers ammo.

Simply put, don't fearmonger or overstate the science, please. And don't buy into manufactured doubt, the trade association's most powerful weapon to induce apathy. What's a trustworthy source? Here's how to know:

Get web-savvy. As a general rule, websites ending in ".gov" and ".edu" are the most credible. Some sites ending with ".org" are also trustworthy, like many of the environmental and public health organizations listed above. Those ending in ".com" are a mixed bag—some are stellar, others not so much. Be very leery of using YouTube, TikTok, or Instagram influencers as a primary news source.

Understand what makes for good journalism. Know that mainstream news publications and the journalists who write for them (unlike social media accounts) are required to uphold basic journalistic standards around reporting (such as giving both sides an opportunity to comment) and fact-checking. An article in a mainstream newspaper or established independent news channel like NPR or PBS is going to be held to a high standard of reporting compared to a TikToker with a few hundred thousand followers. While there is a narrative about the *New York Times* being liberal and the *Wall Street Journal* being conservative, people are conflating the positions of their editorial boards and opinion pages with their reporting. And yes, there is inherent bias in every human, but well-trained journalists—just like well-trained scientists—understand this and work to avoid confirmation bias, aka looking for evidence that supports only preconceived ideas. The First Amendment to the US Constitution protects the freedom of the press, recognizing its importance to an informed electorate and an accountable government. We must work hard to protect the right to free press.

Trust good science. Scientific studies published in peer-reviewed journals are critical, as are the news outlets that regularly demystify the results for the lay audience. Most people can understand the "summary" or "abstract" portion of a study, but it helps to also read news articles about the study results, especially those for which the study authors have been interviewed. Also, know that published studies must include a declaration of competing interest and funding sources at the end. Scroll to the end to see if any corporations or trade groups helped fund the research.

Are you a health professional? I recommend Lara Adler's science-backed course on environmental health geared toward health professionals (laraadler.com).

Follow Environmental Health News (ehn.org), a daily roundup of breaking science and news articles covering environmental health topics. The organization is nonpartisan and nonprofit.

Listen to and support the *Agents of Change in Environmental Justice* podcast, a project founded by Dr. Ami Zota in partnership with *Environmental Health News* and the George Washington University Milken Institute School of Public Health. It features scientific fellows who research the intersection between environmental health and social justice.

Host a book club. The questions at the end of this book will help guide a rich discussion. In the spirit of continuing to build a grassroots movement centered on consumer safety and environmental health, you can play an important role in sharing this book with your friends. During the book club convo, take a pause to all call your senators—strength in numbers!

Be armed with simple responses for dismissers and fearmongers. While you don't want to engage with dismisser content on social media, you may find yourself speaking with a dismissive colleague or family member and have an opportunity to clearly communicate the science of environmental health or to introduce a non-extreme viewpoint. I'm not saying you have to tell your grandpa that his shampoo contains carcinogens at Thanksgiving dinner, but do be alert to natural openings to start a conversation. There are a series of questions I hear time and time again, and if you decide to bring up consumer safety, or this book, you might hear them too. In fact, I really hope you do get FAQs, because we need to be having informed conservations. Here are simple responses to common questions coming from clean-curious folks and skeptics. Remember,

I too was a skeptic, as was Shanna Swan (the scientist from chapter 1 who blew the lid on sperm counts declining by 50 percent worldwide), when first hearing about these issues. You never know who could join us in this fight.

"I don't have time to add one more thing to my to-do list."

"You're right, it's unfair that consumers are carrying the burden and have become our own government agencies. This is all the more reason we need to spend just two minutes to call our elected officials to ask them to support federal and state laws that remove toxic chemicals from our products and communities in the first place. You can cross something off your to-do list: try to buy half the number of things you currently do, which will reduce the amount of toxic chemicals in your home and reduce the overall demand for the production of these chemicals. It's that simple."

"I heard the clean market is all marketing and fearmongering."

"Some players in the market have been touting clean products and not doing the work to actually make them clean, but the reality is that the clean market is needed, and some companies can stand behind claims that their products are safer. Decades' worth of science shows us that many toxic chemicals are still legally allowed in consumer products, and these chemicals have harmful impacts on people who use the products and the communities where these products are made. Just because some people share this information in an unhelpful way, or brands overstate the science, doesn't mean there isn't a real issue. If you can afford to support and shop clean brands, please do. It helps signal to the market that we want and demand safer products."

"My one-hundred-year-old grandma, who smoked, drank heavily, and chased DDT trucks, is still alive and well." "Your point is well taken, and good for her—I'd love to meet your grandma to hear some stories about those DDT trucks. The thing about toxic chemicals is that some people can be impacted while others are not. For example, there are many reasons someone may get cancer in their lifetime—genetics, lifestyle, environmental or workplace exposures. The question is, if we have the ability to remove one of those risk factors, like carcinogens in our products, why wouldn't we? Many people are not as lucky as your grandma."

"I think the bigger problem is climate change." "Climate change is the issue of our lifetime, and this issue of toxic chemicals in consumer products is actually directly related to climate change and a contributor to it. Many of the toxic chemicals, materials, and plastics that are problematic for human health are made from petroleum—a primary source of the greenhouse gas CO_2—in communities right here in the United States. Those communities are traditionally low-income and/or communities of color, and they are being hardest hit by the impacts of these polluting industries."

"The government is already too involved in our lives." "Here's the interesting thing: the lack of government oversight and intervention is exactly how we got into this mess. Take the beauty industry, which was left mostly unregulated for over eighty years. The lack of regulation allowed companies to go unchecked, and they failed to properly police themselves. While our government agencies, like the EPA and FDA, are not perfect, we must remember that they were established to protect us. But they can take action only after Congress has given them the power to do so. It's our responsibility to hold our elected officials accountable to support those agencies and implement strong consumer safety and environmental laws once passed. Our democracy was designed to have us as voters actively engaged in the process.

Summary of Scientific Consensus

"Scientific consensus" is a term used when enough peer-reviewed evidence brings the scientific community into alignment. This concept is particularly helpful to understand when it comes to environmental health research, which many dismissers undercut by stating that the science in this field is "new" and not yet proven. But newly published peer-reviewed research stands on a mountain of related research. Following is a summary of the scientific consensus on chemicals, medical organizations' consensus statements, and positions on the topics explored in this book*:

MEDICAL ORGANIZATIONS' CONSENSUS STATEMENTS

+ American Academy of Pediatrics (professional organization for pediatricians)

+ American College of Obstetricians and Gynecologists (professional organization for OB/GYNs)

+ Endocrine Society (professional organization for endocrinologists): consensus statement from 2009 and 2015

---

* This is not a complete list.

* International Federation of Gynecology and Obstetrics
(professional organization for OB/GYNs): call for removal of
PFAS, heavy metals in prenatal vitamins, and environmental
health and toxic chemical threats

SCIENTIFIC CONSENSUS STATEMENTS

* The San Antonio Statement on Brominated and Chlorinated
Flame Retardants: Impacts and Potential Policy Influence:
A new consensus on reconciling fire safety with the
environmental and health impacts of chemical flame
retardants, signed by more than 220 scientists and physicians
and published in *Environmental Health Perspectives.*

* *Archives of Toxicology* 91, no. 2 (2017): R. Solecki et al.,
"Scientific Principles for the Identification of Endocrine-
Disrupting Chemicals: A Consensus Statement"

* *Endocrine Reviews* 36, no. 6 (2015): A. C. Gore et al., "EDC-2:
The Endocrine Society's Second Scientific Statement on
Endocrine-Disrupting Chemicals"

* *Environmental Science and Pollution Research International*
12, no. 4 (2005): "The Prague Declaration on Endocrine
Disruption"

* *Federal Register* 65, no. 4 (2000): US National Toxicology
Program, "Scientific Peer Review of Low-Dose Studies"

* International Programme on Chemical Safety, World Health
Organization, July 13, 2002: T. Damstra et al., eds., *Global
Assessment of the State-of-the-Science of Endocrine Disruptors*

❋ *Journal of the Endocrine Society* 4, no. 10 (2020): B. Demeneix et al., "Thresholds and Endocrine Disruptors: An Endocrine Society Policy Perspective"

❋ *The Lancet: Diabetes & Endocrinology* 8, no. 8 (2020): C. Kassotis et al., "Endocrine-Disrupting Chemicals: Economic, Regulatory, and Policy Implications"

❋ *The Lancet: Diabetes & Endocrinology* 8, no. 8 (2020): L. Kahn et al., "Endocrine-Disrupting Chemicals: Implications for Human Health"

❋ National Academies Press (1999): National Research Council, *Hormonally-Active Agents in the Environment*

❋ *Nature Reviews: Endocrinology* 16 (2019): M. La Merrill et al., "Consensus on the Key Characteristics of Endocrine-Disrupting Chemicals as a Basis for Hazard Identification"

❋ The Royal Society (June 2000): "Endocrine Disrupting Chemicals (EDCs)"

❋ *Seminars in Reproductive Medicine* 24, no. 3 (2006): Collaborative for Health & Environment, "Vallombrosa Consensus Statement on Environmental Contaminants and Human Fertility Compromise"

❋ *Toxicology and Industrial Health* 14, nos. 1/2 (1998): T. Colborn et al., "Statement from the Work Session on Environmental Endocrine-Disrupting Chemicals: Neural, Endocrine, and Behavioral Effects"

❋ Wingspread Conference (July 1991): "Chemically-Induced Alterations in Sexual Development: The Wildlife/Human

Connection," proceedings from a session at the Wingspread Conference Center, published in *Advances in Modern Environmental Toxicology* 21 (1992)

* Wingspread Conference (December 1993): "Environmentally Induced Alterations in Development: A Focus on Wildlife," proceedings from a session at the Wingspread Conference Center, published in *Environmental Health Perspectives* 103, supp. 4 (1995)

* Wingspread Conference (July 1995): "Chemically-Induced Alterations in Functional Development and Reproduction of Fishes," proceedings from a session at the Wingspread Conference Center, published in 1997 by SETAC Press (see resources section)

* Wingspread Conference (February 1995): "Statement from the Work Session on Chemically-Induced Alterations in the Developing Immune System: The Wildlife/Human Connection," published in *Environmental Health Perspectives* 104, supp. 4 (1996)

* Yokohama International Workshop (December 1999): "Endocrine Disruptors in Living Things" (the Yokohama Consensus Statement)

CATEGORY	PRODUCT*	WHAT TO LOOK FOR
Beauty	Skin care and cosmetics	Products that are EWG Verified or MADE SAFE Verified
	Sunscreen	Mineral-based sunscreen (using sunscreen is still very important!)
	Nail polish	Skip nail polish entirely if you're pregnant. The rest of the time look for brands that are "7" or "10" free. If you like treating yourself to a spa day, opt for a salon with excellent ventilation and wear a mask if having dip nail polish removed.
	Hair	Skip aerosol sprays for dry shampoo and hair spray and opt for pumps instead.
	Perfume and cologne	Look for EWG Verified or formulas with fully disclosed ingredient lists. The safest option? Skip perfume altogether.
	Menstrual products	Look for fragrance-free tampons and pads. Or try something new and purchase a silicone menstrual cup or a reusable pad/menstrual underwear that is OEKO-TEX Certified and PFAS free.
Vitamins	Supplements and protein powder	Shop brands that are Clean Label Project Certified and that publicly share testing.
Kitchen Supplies	Cookware	Buy stainless steel, cast iron, and glass. Use parchment paper on nonstick baking sheets or in an air fryer. Ceramic coatings on pots and pans are nontoxic, but this cookware is an un-sustainable option because the coating wears off quickly— usually within one year.
	Food storage	Opt for glass storage containers and beeswax wrap. Use silicone for snacks. Avoid hard, clear, rigid plastic, even if labeled "BPA-Free."
	Takeout	Minimize takeout food consumption since the packaging is often treated with PFAS.
	Kitchen utensils	Avoid plastic (especially black plastic) and opt for stainless steel or bamboo/hardwood utensils. Silicone is a safer plastic option.

* *Note:* Please check out **heyhilde.com** for brand-specific recommendations.

CATEGORY	PRODUCT*	WHAT TO LOOK FOR
Dry Cleaning		Avoid dry cleaning when possible. Air out dry-cleaned clothes before bringing them into your home, and ask your dry cleaner if they are free from perchlorate and TCE.
Water Filters		Test your tap water prior to investing in a system so you can match your needs to the right one. (Tap Score is the best company). On a budget? Try a water filter that attaches directly to your faucet (great if you're renting!). If you can invest in a larger system, look for one that removes PFAS.
Mattresses		Look for flame-retardant-free brands. Look for a spring mattress over foam.
Clothing		Avoid synthetic 100 percent polyester sports-wear and wrinkle-free shirts. Choose OEKO-TEX Certified when possible. Buying secondhand and at clothing swaps is best. Remember: buy half of what you usually would. PFAS-free rain and performance gear.
Couches		Couches purchased before 2015 have toxic flame retardants in them. If purchased after 2015, look under the couch for a tag to see if it was treated with chemical flame retardants.
Home Goods	Furniture	Purchase furniture that complies with the California formaldehyde law. Read the online comment sections before purchasing to see if customers complain of a strong off-gassing smell.
	Candles	Avoid candles and plug-in air fresheners and sprays, especially if the household includes someone with asthma or respiratory issues. If you are going to use a candle, the safer options are soy-based.
	Shower curtains	Avoid vinyl/PVC. Choose untreated polyester instead.
Flooring	Hard flooring	Avoid vinyl flooring, which can off-gas hormone-disrupting compounds and VOCs. Wet-mop frequently. Opt for wood or linoleum.

* *Note:* Please check out **heyhilde.com** for brand-specific recommendations.

CATEGORY	PRODUCT*	WHAT TO LOOK FOR
Flooring	Carpet	Look for nonrecycled carpet padding. (Recycled foam contains flame retardants from old couches.) Shop with retailers like IKEA and Home Depot, which have banned PFAS from carpets.
	Rugs	Avoid anything labeled with terms similar to "stain resistant." Follow your nose and avoid purchasing a rug with a strong chemical smell (VOCs). Off-gas in a different space if necessary.
Cleaning	Vacuum	Vacuum frequently. Purchase a vacuum with a HEPA filter.
	Cleaners	Use EPA Safer Choice Certified products or vinegar, which kills over 95 percent of viruses and bacteria.
Babies and Kids	Car seats	Opt for flame-retardant-free brands.
	Bottles	Glass is best; polypropylene is a second option. Avoid hard clear rigid plastic bottles, even if they're labeled "BPA-Free."
	Mattresses	Choose flame-retardant free. To avoid being taken in by greenwashing claims, look for the following certifications: GOTS, GOLS, MADE SAFE, and UL GREENGUARD Gold. (Ideally the mattress will have more than one of these certifications.) If possible, find an organic mattress made of cotton, wool, and/or latex.
Food	Produce	Prioritize locally grown, organic, or regenerative produce when possible. Fresh and frozen vegetables are better than canned. Any vegetable and fruit is better than none!
	Meat and dairy	Opt for organic, pasture-raised meats, and dairy (if possible). Also reduce or avoid meat and dairy altogether to lower your carbon footprint.
	Seafood	Aim to consume the "SMASH" fish: sardines, mackerel, anchovies, salmon, and herring. These species have the highest nutritional value and the lowest amount of contaminants. The Seafood Watch app is a great resource for finding sustainable fish.

* *Note:* Please check out **heyhilde.com** for brand-specific recommendations.

BOOK CLUB DISCUSSION QUESTIONS

1. What preconceived notions did you have about the topic of "clean" products, if any, before you read the book? Did you find your opinions changing?

2. We learned about scientists who discovered, in some cases by accident, links between chemicals in our homes and health impacts like cancer and hormone disruption. How did learning about toxic chemicals change the way you think about your approach to health and well-being? Did discovering that there has been a 50 percent drop in sperm counts globally over the last fifty years surprise you?

3. Lindsay Dahl covers the health effects of some chemicals, how they can become global pollutants, and the social justice impacts of these chemicals. Which one of these three topics resonated most with you? Did learning about how chemicals impact people where they are made (Texas) and also where they often end up (Alaska) broaden your thinking around shopping for safer products?

4. Do you consider yourself an activist? How has your stance changed or stayed the same after reading this book?

5. Can you think of a time when you criticized your own political party, or when you held someone you voted for accountable?

6. As we learn in chapter 8, it takes only ten calls a week to convince a senator to pay attention to an issue. Did this number surprise you? Did it change the way you think about the impact of your voice in government? If yes, how so?

7. Dahl talks about the burden on women—and particularly on moms—to carry out the fight for safer products and more robust laws. Do you see the fight for "clean" products as a women's issue? In what ways does it feel similar to under-researched women's health issues? Do you think labeling it a "women's issue" increases or decreases the likelihood of change happening?

8. In chapter 9, Dahl references three categories of consumers: pessimists, dismissers, and pragmatists. Which of these labels, if any, did you most relate to? (No judgment!)

9. In chapter 10, Dahl mentions that we all have a deeply held opinion or two that could use some nuance. What is an opinion you hold that could use a little more exploring?

10. Dahl describes many ways in which you can help in the fight to make consumer products safer. Which of the action items most excite you? Which of them scare you?

ACKNOWLEDGMENTS

Like social movements, writing a book takes a village. My deepest sincere thanks to the following (and many more unnamed):

To my loving husband, who gave me the space and time to write this book over the course of many years. The limited time I had to write this was available only because you made the space for it. You've always been my champion. Thank you.

To my girls, may the world we leave you be a little less toxic than the one we live in today.

To the best writing team a person could ask for: a million thank-yous to Tula Karras, who was with me for every word, and to Jessica Runck for being the writer to get this ten-year vision off the ground.

To my agent, Rebecca Gradinger, who believed in this story's importance and timeliness, even after being told "no" and hearing from so many other agents that it was "too complicated."

To my editors, Libby Burton and Anna Montague at Dey Street, for taking the chance on a first-time author and encouraging me to tell this story through my personal lens.

My deepest gratitude to the following experts who were interviewed for the book and who reviewed relevant chapters for accuracy: Robert Bilott, Dr. Arlene Blum, Pamela Miller, Gregg Renfrew, Representative Jan Schakowsky, Dr. Shanna Swan, Vi Waghiyi, and Dr. Ami Zota.

For the diligent scientific review by Dr. Jennifer McPartland: thank you for pressing me hard to ensure that the science, policy, and politics were accurately portrayed.

To my research team: Parker Johnson, you went above and beyond; thank you for doing the hard, tedious, and important work to make sure the sources and recommendations were buttoned up. In addition, I am grateful for the support of Christine Baumer, Joanna Pambianco, and Lara Adler.

A heartfelt thank-you to the many unnamed leaders who started this movement nearly one hundred years ago and those who carried the torch (many of whom are women): Erin Brokovich, Suzie Canales, Rachel Carson, Vivian Chang, Lois Gibbs, Ruth deForest Lamb, Dolores Huerta, Winona LaDuke, Jean Sloan, Sandra Steingraber, Beverly Wright, and many more.

The following individuals who played an outsize role in passing TSCA reform but were not featured in the book, in addition to the innumerable volunteers and organizations participating in the Safer Chemicals, Healthy Families coalition: Lori Alper, Mike Belliveau, Jose Bravo, Anne Brock, Charlotte Brody, Nancy Buermeyer, Hannah Cary, Barry Cik, Gary Cohen, Ken Cook, Cecil Corbin Mark, Elizabeth Crowe, Kathy Curtis, Richard Denison, Daryl Ditz, Sarah Doll, Tracey Easthope, Emily Enderlee,

Katy Farber, Donna Ferullo, Jan Robinson Flint, Nourbese Flint, Amanda Frayer, Eve Gartner, Kathy Gerwig, Rachel Gibson, Janet Groat, Michael Green, Stephanie Hendricks, Liz Hitchcock, Anne Hulick, Andy Igrejas, Sarah Janssen, Margie Kelly, Rachel Kreigsman, Gretchen Lee Salter, David Levine, Rich Liroff, Cindy Luppi, Roger McFadden, Jennifer McPartland, Ansje Miller, Pamela Miller, Mark Mitchell, Janet Nudelman, Juan Parras, Micaela Preston, Colin Price, Linda Reinstein, Jeanne Rizzo, Judy Robinson, Daniel Rosenberg, Mark Rossi, Mike Schade, Peggy Shepard, Tricia Smith, Gina Solomon, Robert Sussman, Maureen Swanson, Matthew Tejada, Beverley Thorpe, Joel Tickner, Baskut Tuncak, Laurie Valeriano, Sarah Vogel, Vi Waghiyi, Rachelle Wenger, Heather White, and Bobbi Wilding.

A huge thank-you to all the legislative champions, including members of Congress and their staff who helped pass TSCA reform and MoCRA. Their tireless work navigating Hill politics and managing the endless number of stakeholders could easily fill the pages of another book. This gratitude extends to the many silent leaders who sit within federal agencies like the EPA, FDA, CPSC, NIEHS, CDC, and more.

Laurie Valeriano and the team at Toxic Free Future, who took over the management and leadership of the Mind the Store retailer campaign and federal TSCA work. Grateful for learning from you over the decades and ongoing counsel.

My thanks to state legislators who championed consumer safety bills in Minnesota: Senators John Marty, Linda Murphy, and Sandy Rummel and Representatives Karen Clark and Kate Knuth.

To the scientists from whom I've learned over the years: Linda Birnbaum, Richard Clapp, Terry Collins, Kim Harley, Phil Landrigan, Frederick von Saal, Ted Schettler, Ana Soto, Heather Stapleton, Leo Trasande, Laura Vanderberg, David Wallinga, Tracey Woodruff, and many more.

To the mentors and friends from whom I learned in the early years of my career: J. D. Hamilton, Annie Leonard, Stacy Malkan, Michael Nobel, Robyn O'Brien, Kirk Pederson, Sara Rummel, Kathleen Schuler, Peter Starzynski, Jamison Tessneer, and Sarah Uhl.

To the Beautycounter team for taking a chance on me: Gregg Renfrew, for allowing me to use my niche skills with your business; Mia Davis, for the phone call on my way to Shake Shack and the opportunity to leap into the corporate world; Christy Coleman, for teaching me the complexities of formulating cosmetics; and Meaghan Curcio, for being the most talented publicist I know. Thank you to my incredible team and colleagues over the years and the surrounding community of advocates.

To the funding community that had the vision to support long-term investments in environmental health and to those who continue to support the work of the organizations leading the way. A special shout-out to Anita Nager and Ruth Hennig.

To one of my favorite professors at St. Olaf College, Dr. Christopher Brooks, who sent me on a journey to challenge black-and-white, ideological thinking, helped me understand the historical context for the important role critical thinking plays in upholding our democracy, and for introducing me to Václav Havel's work, shaping the future of my career and this book.

A shout-out to the brave authors and journalists who have carefully researched, documented, and exposed many of the deceptive practices by the chemical industry over the years.

To all the teachers at the public interdisciplinary high school I had the privilege of attending, the School of Environmental Studies. The early seeds of my passion for the environment were planted through the school's curriculum and learning environment.

And a final thank-you to my family and my tight inner circle of friends (you know who you are), who have been supporting me along this winding career path since day one.

BIBLIOGRAPHY

Chapter 1

Berkeley Statistics, "About: Shanna Swan." Accessed November 14, 2024, https://statistics.berkeley.edu/150w/shanna-swan.

Blount, B. C., et al., "Levels of Seven Urinary Phthalate Metabolites in a Human Reference Population," *Environmental Health Perspectives* 108, no. 10 (2000): 979–82. https://doi.org/10.1289/ehp.00108979.

Foster, Paul, R. C. Cattley, and E. Mylchreest, "Effects of Di-*n*-butyl Phthalate (DBP) on Male Reproductive Development in the Rat: Implications for Human Risk Assessment," *Food and Chemical Toxicology* 38, no. 1 (2000): S97–99. https://doi.org/10.1016/S0278-6915(99)00128-3.

Ghassabian, Akhgar, et al., "Prenatal Exposure to Common Plasticizers: A Longitudinal Study on Phthalates, Brain Volumetric Measures, and IQ in Youth," *Molecular Psychiatry* 28 (2023): 4814–22. https://doi.org/10.1038/s41380-023-02225-6.

Kazemi, Zahra, et al., "Evaluation of Pollutants in Perfumes, Colognes, and Health Effects on the Consumer: A Systematic Review," *Journal of Environmental Health Science and Engineering* 20 (2022): 589–98. https://doi.org/10.1007/s40201-021-00783-x.

Levine, Hagai, et al., "Temporal Trends in Sperm Count: A Systematic Review and Meta-Regression Analysis," *Human Reproduction Update* 23, no. 6 (2017): 646–59. https://doi.org/10.1093/humupd/dmx022.

Mayo Clinic Staff, "Hypospadias," updated September 12, 2024. https://www.mayoclinic.org/diseases-conditions/hypospadias/symptoms-causes/syc-20355148.

Mendiola, Jaime, et al., "Shorter Anogenital Distance Predicts Poorer Semen Quality in Young Men in Rochester, New York," *Environmental Health Perspectives* 119, no. 7 (2011): 958–63. https://doi.org/10.1289/ehp.1103421.

National Academies of Sciences, Engineering, and Medicine, *Application of Systematic Review Methods in an Overall Strategy for Evaluating Low-Dose Toxicity from Endocrine Active Chemicals: Consensus Report*. National Academies Press (2017), chap. 3. https://doi.org/10.17226/24758.

National Research Council Committee on Hormonally Active Agents in the Environment, *Hormonally Active Agents in the Environment*. National Academies Press (1999). https://www.ncbi.nlm.nih.gov/books/NBK230233/.

Silva, Manori J., et al., "Urinary Levels of Seven Phthalate Metabolites in the US Population from the National Health and Nutrition Examination Survey (NHANES) 1999–2000," *Environmental Health Perspectives* 112, no. 3 (2004): 331–38. https://doi.org/10.1289/ehp.6723.

Swan, Shanna H., interview with the author, September 26, 2023.

Swan, Shanna H., and Willard L. Brown, "Oral Contraceptive Use, Sexual Activity, and Cervical Carcinoma," *American Journal of Obstetrics & Gynecology* 139, no. 1 (1981): P52–27. https://www.ajog.org/article/0002-9378(81)90411-7/abstract.

Swan, Shanna H., with Stacey Colino, *Count Down: How Our Modern World Is Threatening Sperm Counts, Altering Male and Female Reproductive Development, and Imperiling the Future of the Human Race*. Scribner (2020).

Swan, Shanna H., Robin L. Kruse, et al., "Semen Quality in Relation to Biomarkers of Pesticide Exposure," *Environmental Health Perspectives* 111, no. 12 (2003): 1478–74. https://ehp.niehs.nih.gov/doi/10.1289/ehp.6417.

Swan, Shanna H., Katharina M. Main, et al., "Decrease in Anogenital Distance Among Male Infants with Prenatal Phthalate Exposure," *Environmental Health Perspectives* 113, no. 8 (2005): 1056–61. https://doi.org/10.1289/ehp.8100.

Tabuchi, Hiroko. "Two Industry Executives Join E.P.A. to Help Oversee Chemical Rules," *New York Times*, January 22, 2025. https://www.nytimes.com/2025/01/22/climate/epa-chemical-industry-beck-dekleva.html.

CHAPTER 2

Environmental Integrity Project, "Who's Running Trump's EPA?" Accessed November 14, 2024, https://environmentalintegrity.org/trump-watch-epa/whos-running-trumps-epa/.

European Commission, "Permanent Ban of Phthalates: Commission Hails Long-Term Safety for Children's Toys," July 5, 2005. https://ec.europa.eu/commission/presscorner/detail/en/ip_05_838.

Goodman, Julie E., Ernest E. McConnell, et al., "An Updated Weight of the Evidence Evaluation of Reproductive and Developmental Effects of Low Doses of Bisphenol A," *Critical Reviews in Toxicology* 36, no. 5 (2006): 387–457. https://doi.org/10.1080/10408440600758317.

Goodman, Julie E., Raphael J. Witorsch, et al., "Weight-of-Evidence Evaluation of Reproductive and Developmental Effects of Low Doses of Bisphenol A," *Critical Reviews in Toxicology* 39, no. 1 (2009): 1–75. https://doi.org /10.1080/10408440802157839.

Gradient Corporation, "What We Do: Science and Strategies for Health and the Environment." Accessed August 2024, https://gradientcorp.com/.

Heath, David, "Meet the 'Rented White Coats' Who Defend Toxic Chemicals," Center for Public Integrity, February 8, 2016. https://publicintegrity.org /environment/meet-the-rented-white-coats-who-defend-toxic-chemicals/.

Olson, Jeremy, "Ban Sought on Chemicals in Child Products," *Twin Cities Pioneer Press*, February 2008, updated November 14, 2015. https://www .twincities.com/2008/02/25/ban-sought-on-chemicals-in-child-products/.

Open Secrets, "Client Profile: American Chemistry Council," updated October 24, 2024. Accessed November 11, 2024, https://www.opensecrets.org /federal-lobbying/clients/summary?cycle=2024&id=D000000365&name =American+Chemistry+Council.

Open Secrets, "Industry Profile: Chemical & Related Manufacturing," updated October 24, 2024. Acccssed November 11, 2024, https://www.opensecrets .org/federal-lobbying/industries/summary?cycle=2024&id=N13.

Open Secrets, "Our Vision and Mission: Inform, Empower & Advocate." Accessed November 11, 2024, https://www.opensecrets.org/about.

US Consumer Product Safety Commission, "RC2 Corp. Recalls Various Thomas & Friends™ Wooden Railway Toys Due to Lead Poisoning Hazard," June 13, 2007. https://www.cpsc.gov/Recalls/2007/rc2-corp-recalls-various-thomas -friends-wooden-railway-toys-due-to-lead-poisoning.

US Environmental Protection Agency, "Protect Your Family from Sources of Lead," updated December 6, 2024. https://www.epa.gov/lead/protect-your -family-sources-lead.

CHAPTER 3

Alexander, Barbara M., and Stuart C. Baxter, "Flame-Retardant Contamination of Firefighter Personal Protective Clothing—A Potential Health Risk for Firefighters," *Journal of Occupational and Environmental Hygiene* 13, no. 9 (2016): D148–55. https://doi.org/10.1080/15459624.2016.1183016.

Blum, Arlene, interview with the author, October 10, 2023.

Blum, Arlene, and Bruce N. Ames, "Flame-Retardant Additives as Possible Cancer Hazards," *Science* 195, no. 4273 (1977): 17–23. https://doi.org /10.1126/science.831254.

Butt, Craig M., et al., "Metabolites of Organophosphate Flame Retardants and 2-Ethylhexyl Tetrabromobenzoate in Urine from Paired Mothers and Toddlers," *Environmental Science & Technology* 48, no. 17 (2014): 10432–38. https://doi.org/10.1021/es5025299.

California Department of Consumer Affairs, Bureau of Household Goods and Services, "Technical Bulletin 117: Residential Upholstered Furniture Standard Fact Sheet." Accessed November 17, 2024, https://bhgs.dca.ca.gov /industry/tb_117_faq_sheet.pdf.

California Professional Firefighters, "FF Cancer Risk Cited in Bid to Reform Flame Retardant Standard," updated August 4, 2020. https://legacy.cpf.org /go/cpf/news-and-events/news/ff-cancer-risk-cited-in-bid-to-reform-flame -retardant-standard/index.html.

Callaghan, Patricia, and Sam Roe, "Fear Fans Flames for Chemical Makers," *Chicago Tribune*, May 6, 2012. https://www.chicagotribune. com/2012/05/06/fear-fans-flames-for-chemical-makers-3/.

Moretto, Marin, "Exposure to Flame Retardant Chemicals Means Firefighters Face Higher Cancer Risk than Previously Thought," *Bangor Daily News*, May 13, 2013. https://www.sffcpf.org/firefighters-face-higher-cancer -risk/.

National Commission on Fire Prevention and Control, *America Burning: The Report of the National Commission on Fire Prevention and Control*, May 1973. https://www.usfa.fema.gov/downloads/pdf/publications/fa -264.pdf.

Russell, Christine, "Science Leaders Fear 'Irreversible Damage' from Budget Cuts," *Washington Post*, October 27, 1981. https://www.washingtonpost .com/archive/politics/1981/10/28/science-leaders-fear-irreversible-damage -from-budget-cuts/5950b676-147d-46ee-be86-c71e84eedf96/.

Slater, Dashka, "How Dangerous Is Your Couch?," *New York Times Magazine*, September 6, 2012. https://www.nytimes.com/2012/09/09/magazine /arlene-blums-crusade-against-household-toxins.html.

Vuong, Ann M., et al., "Flame Retardants and Neurodevelopment: An Updated Review of Epidemiological Literature," *Environmental Epidemiology* 7, no. 4 (2020): 220–36. https://doi.org/10.1007/s40471-020-00256-z.

Way, Ron, "Pawlenty Digs Deeper into a Hole with Veto Reasoning," *MinnPost*, May 14, 2008. https://www.minnpost.com/environment/2008/05/ pawlenty-digs-deeper-hole-veto-reasoning/.

CHAPTER 4

Air Alliance Houston, "Houston's Dirty Dozen: A Report on the Top Industrial Air Polluters," July 2024. https://airalliancehouston.org/wp-content/uploads/2024/07/AAH-Dirty-Dozen-Report.pdf.

American Lung Association, "Texas: Galveston: What's the State of Your Air?" Accessed August 14, 2024, https://www.lung.org/research/sota/city-rankings/states/texas/galveston.

Aulds, T. J., "A Quick Guide to the Major Industrial Players in Texas City," *Galveston Daily News*, April 20, 2013. https://www.galvnews.com/profiles/business-industry/a-quick-guide-to-the-major-industrial-players-in-texas-city/article_5214cc1a-a867-11e2-852f-001a4bcf6878.html.

Baurick, Tristan, Lylla Younes, and Joan Meiners, "Polluter's Paradise: Welcome to 'Cancer Alley,' Where Toxic Air Is About to Get Worse," *ProPublica*, October 30, 2019. https://www.propublica.org/article/welcome-to-cancer-alley-where-toxic-air-is-about-to-get-worse.

Bethel, Heidi L., et al., "A Closer Look at Air Pollution in Houston: Identifying Priority Health Risks," US Environmental Protection Agency, June 2006. https://www3.epa.gov/ttnchie1/conference/ei16/session6/bethel.pdf.

Byrne, Samuel C., "Persistent Organic Pollutants in the Arctic," Alaska Community Action on Toxics, May 2009. https://www.akaction.org/wp-content/uploads/POPs_in_the_Arctic_ACAT_May_2009-2.pdf.

Campaign for Healthier Solutions, "Toxic Chemicals in Dollar Store Products: 2022 Report," August 2022. https://www.ecocenter.org/sites/default/files/2022-08/Toxic%20Chemicals%20in%20Dollar%20Store%20Products%202022%20Report.pdf.

Clark-Leach, Gabriel, et al., "Breakdowns in Enforcement: Texas Rarely Penalizes Industry for Illegal Air Pollution Released During Malfunctions and Maintenance," Environmental Integrity Project, July 7, 2017. https://environmentamerica.org/texas/wp-content/uploads/2017/07/Breakdowns-in-Enforcement-Report-2.pdf.

Dreier, Hanna, "Alone and Exploited, Migrant Children Work Brutal Jobs Across the US," *New York Times*, February 25, 2023, updated February 28, 2023. https://www.nytimes.com/2023/02/25/us/unaccompanied-migrant-child-workers-exploitation.html.

Environmental Defense Fund, "Finding Pollution—and Who It Impacts Most—in Houston," June 3, 2020. https://www.edf.org/airqualitymaps/houston/findings.

Environmental Integrity Project, "56 Refineries with Benzene Readings at the Fenceline Above Potential Health Threat Level in 2021," May 2022.

https://environmentalintegrity.org/wp-content/uploads/2022/05/Updated -health-threat-level-table.pdf.

Fitzgerald, E. F., et al., "Fish Consumption and Breast Milk PCB Concentrations Among Mohawk Women at Akwesasne," *American Journal of Epidemiology* 148, no. 2 (1998): 164–72. https://doi.org/10.1093/oxfordjournals.aje .a009620.

Galveston-Houston Association for Smog Prevention, "Mercury in Galveston and Houston Fish: Contamination by Neurotoxin Places Children at Risk," October 2004. https://airalliancehouston.org/wp-content/uploads/2019/09 /GHASP_Mercury.pdf.

Hirschman, Charles, and Elizabeth Mogford, "Immigration and the American Industrial Revolution from 1880 to 1920," *Social Science Research* 38, no. 4 (2009): 897–920. https://doi.org/10.1016/j.ssresearch.2009.04.001.

Hoover, Elizabeth, et al., "Indigenous Peoples of North America: Environmental Exposures and Reproductive Justice," *Environmental Health Perspectives* 120, no. 12 (2012): 1645–49. https://doi.org/10.1289/ehp.1205422.

House Energy and Commerce Committee. "Representatives." Accessed August 14, 2024, https://energycommerce.house.gov/representatives.

Korn, Jennifer, and Marie Barbier, "A Look Back at Every iPhone Ever," *CNN Business*, September 11, 2023. https://www.cnn.com/2023/09/11/tech /iphone-timeline/index.html.

Macdonald, R. W., et al., "Contaminants in the Canadian Arctic: 5 Years of Progress in Understanding Sources, Occurrence, and Pathways," *Science of the Total Environment* 245, nos. 2/3 (2000): 93–234. https://doi.org /10.1016/S0048-9697(00)00434-4.

Mazurek, Jacek M., et al., "Malignant Mesothelioma Mortality: United States, 1999–2015," *Morbidity and Mortality Weekly Report* 66, no. 8 (2017): 214–18. http://doi.org/10.15585/mmwr.mm6608a3.

Miller, Pamela, interview with the author, November 7, 2023.

Miller, Pamela K., et al., "Community-Based Participatory Research Projects and Policy Engagement to Protect Environmental Health on St. Lawrence Island, Alaska," *International Journal of Circumpolar Health* 72, no. 1 (2013). https://doi.org/10.3402/ijch.v72i0.21656.

Mogensen, Ulla B., et al., "Breastfeeding as an Exposure Pathway for Perfluorinated Alkylates," *Environmental Science & Technology* 49, no. 17 (2015): 10466–73. https://doi.org/10.1021/acs.est.5b02237.

National Oceanic and Atmospheric Administration, National Ocean Service, "What Are PCBs?," updated June 16, 2024. https://oceanservice.noaa.gov /facts/pcbs.html.

Parras, Juan, "Oral History Interview with Juan Parras," interview by Sandra Enriquez and Samantha Rodriguez, "Civil Rights in Black and Brown" collection, TCU Mary Couts Burnett Library, June 2016. https://texashistory.unt.edu/ark:/67531/metapth987501/m1/.

Petras, Sarah B., "State of the Science: Children's Environmental Health in Alaska and the Circumpolar North—Protecting Children at the Top of the World," Children's Environmental Health Summit, June 2017. https://www.akaction.org/wp-content/uploads/WHOLE-WHOLE-CEH-6-28-17.pdf.

Press, Eyal, "America Runs on 'Dirty Work' and Moral Inequity," *New York Times*, August 13, 2021. https://www.nytimes.com/2021/08/13/opinion/us-dirty-work.html.

Robinson, Kelly J., et al., "Persistent Organic Pollutant Burden, Experimental POP Exposure, and Tissue Properties Affect Metabolic Profiles of Blubber from Gray Seal Pups," *Environmental Science & Technology* 52, no. 22 (2018): 13523–34. https://doi.org/10.1021/acs.est.8b04240.

Saxton, Dvera I., et al., "Environmental Health and Justice and the Right to Research: Institutional Review Board Denials of Community-Based Chemical Biomonitoring of Breast Milk," *Environmental Health* 14, no. 90 (2015). https://doi.org/10.1186/s12940-015-0076-x.

Scrudato, R. J., et al., "Contaminants at Arctic Formerly Used Defense Sites," *Journal of Local and Global Health Science* 2012, no. 1 (2012). http://doi.org/10.5339/jlghs.2012.2.

Symanski, Elaine, et al., "Air Toxics and Early Childhood Acute Lymphocytic Leukemia in Texas: A Population Based Case Control Study," *Environmental Health* 15, no. 70 (2016). https://doi.org/10.1186/s12940-016-0154-8.

Target Corporation, "Responsible Resource Use: Chemicals." Accessed November 18, 2024, https://corporate.target.com/sustainability-governance/responsible-resource-use/chemicals.

Terrell, Kimberly A., and Gianna St. Julien, "Air Pollution Is Linked to Higher Cancer Rates Among Black or Impoverished Communities in Louisiana," *Environmental Research Letters* 17, no. 1 (2022). http://doi.org/10.1088/1748-9326/ac4360.

Texas Environmental Justice Advocacy Services, "Chemical Security." Accessed August 14, 2024, https://www.tejasbarrios.org/chemical-security.

Tsukimori, Kiyomi, et al., "Long-Term Effects of Polychlorinated Biphenyls and Dioxins on Pregnancy Outcomes in Women Affected by the Yusho Incident," *Environmental Health Perspectives* 116, no. 5 (2008): 626–30. https://doi.org/10.1289/ehp.10686.

US Census Bureau, "Quick Facts: Galveston City, Texas," Census Population, April 1, 2010. Accessed November 18, 2024, https://www.census.gov /quickfacts/fact/table/galvestoncitytexas/PST045222.

US Department of Labor, Occupational Safety and Health Administration, "Ethylene Oxide," *OSHA Fact Sheet*, 2002. Accessed November 18, 2024, https://www.osha.gov/sites/default/files/publications/ethylene-oxide -factsheet.pdf.

US Environmental Protection Agency, *America's Children and the Environment*, 3rd ed., January 2013. https://www.epa.gov/sites/default/files/2015-06/ documents/ace3_2013.pdf.

US Environmental Protection Agency, "Asbestos Laws and Regulations," updated December 31, 2024. Accessed November 11, 2024, https://www.epa.gov /asbestos/asbestos-laws-and-regulations.

US Environmental Protection Agency, "EPA Releases First Major Update to Chemicals List in 40 Years," February 19, 2019. https://www.epa.gov /newsreleases/epa-releases-first-major-update-chemicals-list-40-years.

US Environmental Protection Agency, "Learn About Polychlorinated Biphenyls," updated October 17, 2024. https://www.epa.gov/pchs/learn-about -polychlorinated-biphenyls#healtheffects.

US Environmental Protection Agency, "Summary of the Toxic Substances Control Act," updated September 9, 2024. Accessed November 11, 2024, https://www.epa.gov/laws-regulations/summary-toxic-substances-control -act.

US Environmental Protection Agency, "Toxics Release Inventory (TRI) Program," updated December 26, 2024. Accessed November 18, 2024, https://www.epa.gov/toxics-release-inventory-tri-program.

Waghiyi, Viola, interview with the author, November 7, 2023.

Whitworth, Kristina W., Elaine Symanski, and Ann L. Coker, "Childhood Lymphohematopoietic Cancer Incidence and Hazardous Air Pollutants in Southeast Texas, 1995–2004," *Environmental Health Perspectives* 116, no. 11 (2008): 1576–80. https://doi.org/10.1289/ehp.11593.

CHAPTER 5

Agency for Toxic Substances and Disease Registry, "Fast Facts: PFAS in the US Population," updated November 12, 2024. https://www.atsdr.cdc.gov/pfas/ data-research/facts-stats/?CDC_AAref_Val=https://www.atsdr.cdc.gov/pfas/ health-effects/us-population.html.

Bilott, Robert, interview with the author, September 5, 2023.

Bilott, Robert, *Exposure: Poisoned Water, Corporate Greed, and One Lawyer's Twenty-Year Battle Against DuPont*. Atria (2019).

Centers for Disease Control and Prevention, "National Report on Human Exposure to Environmental Chemicals: Serum Perfluorooctanoic Acid (PFOA) (2011–2018)." https://www.cdc.gov/exposurereport/report/pdf /cgroup23_LBXPFA1_2011-p.pdf.

Cohen, Nathan J., et al., "Exposure to Perfluoroalkyl Substances and Women's Fertility Outcomes in a Singaporean Population-Based Preconception Cohort," *Science of the Total Environment* 873 (2023). https://doi.org /10.1016/j.scitotenv.2023.162267.

Gaber, Nadia, Lisa Bero, and Tracey J. Woodruff, "The Devil They Knew: Chemical Documents Analysis of Industry Influence on PFAS Science," *Annals of Global Health* 89, no. 1 (2023): 37. https://doi.org/10.5334 /aogh.4013.

Interstate Technology Regulatory Council, "History and Use of Per- and Polyfluoroalkyl Substances (PFAS) Found in the Environment," updated September 2023. https://pfas-1.itrcweb.org/wp-content/uploads/2020/10 /history_and_use_508_2020Aug_Final.pdf.

Lerner, Sharon, "The Teflon Toxin: DuPont and the Chemistry of Deception," *The Intercept*, August 11, 2015. https://theintercept.com/2015/08/11 /dupont-chemistry-deception/.

PFAS-TOX Database, updated August 9, 2022. https://pfastoxdatabase.org/.

Rich, Nathaniel, "The Lawyer Who Became DuPont's Worst Nightmare," *New York Times Magazine*, January 2016. https://www.nytimes.com /2016/01/10/magazine/the-lawyer-who-became-duponts-worst-nightmare .html.

Spanne, Autumn, "What Are PFAS?" *Environmental Health News*, February 15, 2022. https://www.ehn.org/what-are-pfas-2656619391.html.

US Environmental Protection Agency, "Consent Agreement and Proposed Final Order to Resolve DuPont's Alleged Failure to Submit Substantial Risk Information Under the Toxic Substances Control Act (TSCA) and Failure to Submit Data Requested Under the Resource Conservation and Recovery Act," December 14, 2005. https://www.epa.gov/sites/default/files/2013-08 /documents/eabmemodupontpfoasettlement121405.pdf.

US Environmental Protection Agency, "Risk Management for Per- and Polyfluoroalkyl Substances (PFAS) Under TSCA," updated October 16, 2024. https://www.epa.gov/assessing-and-managing-chemicals-under-tsca /risk-management-and-polyfluoroalkyl-substances-pfas.

Zhan, Wenqiang, et al., "Environmental Exposure to Emerging Alternatives of Per- and Polyfluoroalkyl Substances and Polycystic Ovarian Syndrome in

Women Diagnosed with Infertility: A Mixture Analysis," *Environmental Health Perspectives* 131, no. 5 (2023). https://doi.org/10.1289/EHP11814.

CHAPTER 6

Agency for Toxic Substances and Disease Registry, "Per- and Polyfluoroalkyl Substances (PFAS) and Your Health: PFAS in the US Population," updated November 14, 2024. https://www.atsdr.cdc.gov/pfas/data-research/facts -stats/?CDC_AAref_Val=https://www.atsdr.cdc.gov/pfas/health-effects/us -population.html.

ChemSafetyPRO, "Overview of Chemical Regulations in Korea," 2015. https://www.chemsafetypro.com/Topics/Korea/Overview_of_Chemical _Regulations_in_Korea.html.

Denison, Richard, "The Truth Will Out: Chemical Industry's Deceptive Tactics Are Eventually Exposed," Environmental Defense Fund, May 6, 2012. https://blogs.edf.org/health/2012/05/06/the-truth-will-out-chemical -industrys-deceptive-tactics-are-eventually-exposed/.

European Union, EUR-Lex, "Consolidated Text: Regulation (EC) No. 1223/2009 of the European Parliament and of the Council of 30 November 2009 on Cosmetic Products (Recast)," updated April 24, 2024. https://eur-lex.europa.eu/legal-content/EN/TXT/?uri=CELEX:02009 R1223-20190813.

Fenton, Suzanne E., et al., "Per- and Polyfluoroalkyl Substance Toxicity and Human Health Review: Current State of Knowledge and Strategies for Informing Future Research," *Environmental Toxicology and Chemistry* 40, no. 3 (2020): 606–30. https://doi.org/10.1002/etc.4890.

Huang, Zongyun, William P. Fish, and Jason Sweeney, "Leaching Rate of Diethylhexyl Phthalate (DEHP) from PVC Containers with IV Administrated Lipid Nanoparticle Formulations," *Journal of Drug Delivery Science and Technology* 80 (2023). https://doi.org/10.1016/j.jddst.2023.104160.

Iallonardo, Tony, "Poll Finds Americans Very Concerned About Exposure to Toxic Chemicals," Toxic-Free FUTURE, November 12, 2009. https:// toxicfreefuture.org/blog/poll-finds-americans-very-concerned-about -exposure-to-toxic-chemicals-2/.

Japan Ministry of the Environment, Environmental Health Department, Chemical Evaluation Office, "Management of Chemicals in Japan," October 2014. https://www.env.go.jp/content/900451424.pdf.

Ko, Elizabeth, and Eve Glazier, "Eating Microwave Popcorn Increases the Level of PFAS in Body," UCLA Health, August 5, 2022. https://www.uclahealth .org/news/article/eating-microwave-popcorn-increases-the-level-of-pfas-in -body.

Maslin Nir, Sarah, "Perfect Nails, Poisoned Workers," *New York Times Magazine*, May 8, 2015. https://www.nytimes.com/2015/05/11/nyregion/nail-salon -workers-in-nyc-face-hazardous-chemicals.html.

National Academies of Sciences, Engineering, and Medicine, *Guidance on PFAS Exposure, Testing, and Clinical Follow-Up*, National Academies Press (2022), chap. 3. https://www.ncbi.nlm.nih.gov/books/NBK584690/.

NYU Langone Health, "NYU Grossman School of Medicine: Leonardo Trasande, MD, MPP." https://med.nyu.edu/faculty/leonardo-trasande.

Siegel, Miriam R., et al., "Maternal Occupation as a Nail Technician or Hairdresser During Pregnancy and Birth Defects: National Birth Defects Prevention Study, 1997–2011," *Occupational & Environmental Medicine* 79, no. 1 (2022). https://doi.org/10.1136/oemed-2021-107561.

Toxicology Excellence for Risk Assessment, "2012 Project Time by Sponsor," 2012. https://tera.org/about/2012_Sponsors.pdf.

Toxicology Excellence for Risk Assessment, "Annual Funding Sources." Accessed November 14, 2024, https://tera.org/about/FundingSources.html.

University of Massachusetts at Lowell, "Richard Clapp, D.Sc." Accessed August 16, 2024, https://www.uml.edu/research/lowell-center/about/team /clapp-richard.aspx.

CHAPTER 7

Ceballos, Diana M., et al., "Biological and Environmental Exposure Monitoring of Volatile Organic Compounds Among Nail Technicians in the Greater Boston Area," *Indoor Air* 29, no. 4 (2019): 539–50. https://doi.org/10.1111 /ina.12564.

Columbia University Medical Center, Department of Dermatology, "Studies on Hair Loss (Alopecia) Associated with Use of Cosmetic Hair Products and Ingredients in These Products: Final Report," September 2022. https://www .fda.gov/media/174193/download?attachment.

Congress.gov, "H.R. 1385: To Amend Title VI of the Federal Food, Drug, and Cosmetic Act to Ensure the Safe Use of Cosmetics, and for Other Purposes," 113th Cong. (2013–2014), 1st sess. https://www.congress.gov/bill/113th -congress/house-bill/1385/text#toc-H553A11A3AE184847BE49E1959 0D28006.

Draelos, Zoe Diana, "Cosmeceuticals: Undefined, Unclassified, and Unregulated," *Clinics in Dermatology* 27, no. 5 (2009): 431434. https://doi.org/10.1016 /j.clindermatol.2009.05.005.

Gasch, Alice T., "Lash Lure and Paraphenylenediamine: Toxic Beauty Past and Present," American Academy of Ophthalmology, November 2, 2017.

https://www.aao.org/lifetime-engaged-ophthalmologist/perspective/article/lash-lure-paraphenylenediamine-toxic-beauty.

Ghazipura, Marya, et. al., "Exposure to Benzophenone-3 and Reproductive Toxicity: A Systematic Review of Human and Animal Studies," *Reproductive Toxicology* 73 (2017): 175–83. https://doi.org/10.1016/j.reprotox.2017.08.015.

Goossens, An, and Olivier Aerts, "Contact Allergy to and Allergic Contact Dermatitis from Formaldehyde and Formaldehyde Releasers: A Clinical Review and Update," *Contact Dermatitis*, 87, no. 1 (2022): 20–27. https://doi.org/10.1111/cod.14089.

Holman, Jordyn, and Maureen Farrell, "How a Distinctive Beauty Brand Fell Apart, Sinking Almost $700 Million with It," *New York Times Magazine*, July 10, 2024. https://www.nytimes.com/2024/07/10/business/beautycounter-carlyle-gregg-renfrew.html.

International Agency for Research on Cancer, World Health Organization, "IARC Monographs Evaluate the Carcinogenicity of Talc and Acrylonitrile: *IARC Monographs* Volume 136: Questions and Answers (Q&A)," July 5, 2024. https://www.iarc.who.int/wp-content/uploads/2024/07/QA-Mono-Vol136.pdf.

Kadry Taher, Mohamed, et al., "Critical Review of the Association Between Perineal Use of Talc Powder and Risk of Ovarian Cancer," *Reproductive Toxicology* 90 (2019): 88–101. https://doi.org/10.1016/j.reprotox.2019.08.015.

Lam, Clinton, and Pretti Patel, "Food, Drug, and Cosmetic Act," updated July 31, 2023, in *StatPearls* (StatPearls Publishing, 2024). https://www.ncbi.nlm.nih.gov/books/NBK585046/.

Lamb, Ruth deForest, *American Chamber of Horrors: The Truth About Food and Drugs*. Farrar & Rinehart (1936).

MarketResearch.biz, "Clean Beauty Market Projected to Grow at 16.65% CAGR by 2033, North America to Be the Dominant Region," January 23, 2024. https://finance.yahoo.com/news/clean-beauty-market-projected-grow-073500195.html?guccounter=1.

Material Properties, "Polyoxymethylene." Accessed September 16, 2024, https://material-properties.org/polyoxymethylene/.

Mayo, Anna, "2023 Glow-Up: The Future of Clean Beauty," NielsenIQ, October 18, 2021. https://nielseniq.com/global/en/insights/analysis/2021/2030-glow-up-the-future-of-clean-beauty/.

National Toxicology Program, *Report on Carcinogens*, 15th ed., US Department of Health and Human Services, December 2021. https://doi.org/10.22427/NTP-OTHER-1003.

Petruzzi, Dominique, "Natural Household Cleaners Market Value in the US from 2015 to 2025," Statista, February 22, 2024. https://www.statista.com /statistics/1064605/natural-household-cleaners-market-value-us/.

Renfrew, Gregg, interview with the author, September 20, 2024.

Sephora, "Clean at Sephora Skincare." Accessed November 14, 2024, https:// www.sephora.com/beauty/clean-skincare-products?icid2=cleanplanetaware _skincare_childlink_linkex_fy243237_cleanplanet0424.

Straits Research, "Natural Household Cleaners Market Size, Share, and Trends Analysis Report by Product . . . by Application . . . by Distribution Channel . . . and by Region . . . Forecasts 2024–2032," August 7, 2024. https://straitsresearch.com/report/natural-household-cleaners-market.

Swann, John P., "FDA's Origin," US Food and Drug Administration, updated February 1, 2018. https://www.fda.gov/about-fda/changes-science-law-and -regulatory-authorities/fdas-origin.

Tchounwou, Paul B., Clement G. Yedjou, Anita K. Patlolla, and Dwanye J. Sutton, "Heavy Metals Toxicity and the Environment," *Molecular, Clinical, and Environmental Toxicology* 101 (2012): 133–64. https://doi .org/10.1007/978-3-7643-8340-4_6.

US Environmental Protection Agency, "Ground Water and Drinking Water: Basic Information About Lead in Drinking Water," updated November 21, 2024. https://www.epa.gov/ground-water-and-drinking-water/basic -information-about-lead-drinking-water#regs.

US Environmental Protection Agency, "What EPA Is Doing to Reduce Mercury Pollution, and Exposures to Mercury," updated July 11, 2024. https://www .epa.gov/mercury/what-epa-doing-reduce-mercury-pollution-and-exposures -mercury.

US Food and Drug Administration, "Cosmetic Products: Hair Dyes," updated October 15, 2024. https://www.fda.gov/cosmetics/cosmetic-products/hair -dyes#safety.

US Food and Drug Administration, "Mercury Poisoning Linked to Skin Products," updated December 21, 2022. https://www.fda.gov/consumers/consumer -updates/mercury-poisoning-linked-skin-products.

US Food and Drug Administration, "Prohibited and Restricted Ingredients in Cosmetics," updated February 25, 2022. https://www.fda.gov/cosmetics /cosmetics-laws-regulations/prohibited-restricted-ingredients-cosmetics #prohibited.

Vega, Nicolas, and Lauren Shamo, "How a 40-Ounce Cup Turned Stanley into a $750 Million a Year Business," CNBC, December 23, 2023. https://www .cnbc.com/2023/12/23/how-a-40-ounce-cup-turned-stanley-into-a-750 -million-a-year-business.html.

Vieira de Freitas Netto, Sebastião, Marcos Felipe Falcão Sobral, Ana Regina Bezerra Ribeiro, and Gleibson Robert da Luz Soares, "Concepts and Forms of Greenwashing: A Systematic Review," *Environmental Sciences Europe* 32, no. 19 (2020). https://doi.org/10.1186/s12302-020-0300-3.

CHAPTER 8

Bariani, Maria, et al., "The Role of Endocrine-Disrupting Chemicals in Uterine Fibroid Pathogenesis," *Current Opinion in Endocrinology, Diabetes, and Obesity* 27, no. 6 (2020): 380–87. https://doi.org/10.1097/med .0000000000000578.

Branch, Francesca, Tracey J. Woodruff, Susanna D. Mitro, and Ami R. Zota, "Vaginal Douching and Racial/Ethnic Disparities in Phthalates Exposures Among Reproductive-Aged Women: National Health and Nutrition Examination Survey 2001–2004," *Environmental Health* 14, no. 57 (2015). https://doi.org/10.1186/s12940-015-0043-6.

Burdeau, Jordan A., et al., "First Trimester Plasma Per- and Polyfluoroalkyl Substances (PFAS) and Blood Pressure Trajectories Across the Second and Third Trimesters of Pregnancy," *Environment International* 186 (2024). https://doi.org/10.1016/j.envint.2024.108628.

California Legislative Information, "AB-2775 Professional Cosmetics: Labeling Requirements," September 17, 2018. https://leginfo.legislature.ca.gov/faces /billTextClient.xhtml?bill_id=201720180AB2775.

Chang, Che-Jung, et al., "Use of Straighteners and Other Hair Products and Incident Uterine Cancer," *Journal of the National Cancer Institute* 114, no. 12 (2022): 1636–45. https://doi.org/10.1093/jnci/djac165.

Congress.gov, "H.R. 4040, Consumer Product Safety Improvement Act of 2008," 110th Cong. (2007–2008), August 14, 2008. https://www.congress .gov/bill/110th-congress/house-bill/4040.

Durgam, Srinivas, and Elena Page, "Formaldehyde Exposures During Brazilian Blowout Hair Smoothing Treatment at a Hair Salon—Ohio," *CDC Workplace Safety and Health*, November 2011. https://www.cdc.gov/niosh /hhe/reports/pdfs/2011-0014-3147.pdf.

Llanos, Adana A. M., et al., "Hair Product Use and Breast Cancer Risk Among African American and White Women," *Oxford Journals: Carcinogenesis* 39, no. 9 (2017): 883–92. https://doi.org/10.1093/carcin/bgx060.

Pierce, J. S., et al., "Characterization of Formaldehyde Exposure Resulting from the Use of Four Professional Hair Straightening Products," *Journal of Occupational and Environmental Hygiene* 8, no. 11 (2011): 686–99. https:// doi.org/10.1080/15459624.2011.626259.

Preston, Emma V., et al., "Early-Pregnancy Plasma Per- and Polyfluoroalkyl Substance (PFAS) Concentrations and Hypertensive Disorders of Pregnancy in the Project Viva Cohort," *Environmental International* 165 (2022). https://doi.org/10.1016/j.envint.2022.107335.

Schakowsky, Janice, interview with the author, September 29, 2023.

Siegel, Miriam R., et al., "Maternal Occupation as a Nail Technician or Hairdresser During Pregnancy and Birth Defects, National Birth Defects Prevention Study, 1997–2011," *Occupational & Environmental Medicine* 79, no. 1 (2022). https://doi.org/10.1136/oemed-2021 -107561.

United States Congresswoman Jan Schakowsky, "About Jan." Accessed September 18, 2024, https://schakowsky.house.gov/about.

US Environmental Protection Agency, "Asbestos Laws and Regulations," updated December 31, 2024. https://www.epa.gov/asbestos/asbestos-laws-and -regulations.

Zota, Ami, interview with the author, November 1, 2023.

Zota, Ami R., and Bhavna Shamasunder, "The Environmental Injustice of Beauty: Framing Chemical Exposures from Beauty Products as a Health Disparities Concern," *American Journal of Obstetrics and Gynecology* 217, no. 4 (2017): 418.e1–6. https://doi.org/10.1016/j.ajog .2017.07.020.

Zota, Ami R., et al., "Environmental Phthalates Exposure and Measures of Uterine Fibroid Size Among a Racially Diverse Population of Premenopausal Women," *ISEE Conference Abstracts* 2018, no. 1 (2018). https://doi.org/10 .1289/isesisee.2018.S03.02.17.

CHAPTER 9

Baker, Stephanie Alice, "Alt. Health Influencers: How Wellness Culture and Web Culture Have Been Weaponized to Promote Conspiracy Theories and Far-Right Extremism During the COVID-19 Pandemic," *European Journal of Cultural Studies* 25, no. 1 (2022). https://doi.org/10.1177 /13675494211062623.

Congress.gov, "H.R. 2617: Consolidated Appropriations Act," 117th Cong. (2021–2022), December 23, 2022. https://www.congress.gov/bill/117th -congress/house-bill/2617.

Daedal Research, *Clean Beauty Market: Analysis by Product Type . . . by Distribution Channel . . . by Region Size and Trends with Impact of COVID-19 and Forecast Up to 2028*, February 2023. https://www .researchandmarkets.com/reports/5734363/clean-beauty-market-analysis

-product-type-skin#:~:text=The%20global%20clean%20beauty%20 market%20was%20valued%20at,has%20all%20the%20ingredients%20 mentioned%20in%20the%20labeling.

Eberle, Carolyn E., Dale P. Sandler, Kyla W. Taylor, and Alexandra J. White, "Hair Dye and Chemical Straightener Use and Breast Cancer Risk in a Large US Population of Black and White Women," *International Journal of Cancer* 147, no. 2 (2019): 383–91. https://doi.org/10.1002/ijc.32738.

Ferreira Caceres, Maria Mercedes, et al., "The Impact of Misinformation on the COVID-19 Pandemic," *AIMS Public Health* 9, no. 2 (2022): 262–77. https://doi.org/10.3934/publichealth.2022018.

National Oceanic and Atmospheric Administration, National Weather Service, "Clouds and Contrails." Accessed November 18, 2024, https://www .weather.gov/fgz/CloudsContrails.

Personal Care Products Council, "Where Innovation Meets Inspiration" (home page). Accessed September 14, 2024, https://www.personalcarecouncil.org/.

Timsit, Annabelle, "Herbal Essences, Pantene Aerosol Products Recalled over Concerns About Cancer-Causing Chemical," *Washington Post*, December 21, 2021. https://www.washingtonpost.com/nation/2021/12/21/procter gamble-recall-dry-shampoo/.

US Senate Committee on Health, Education, Labor, and Pension (HELP), "Exploring Current Practices in Cosmetic Development and Safety," hearing testimony of Beth Lange Jonas, PhD, Chief Scientist, Personal Care Products Council, September 22, 2016. https://www.help.senate.gov/imo /media/doc/Jonas3.pdf.

CHAPTER 10

Angrand, Ruth C., Geoffrey Collins, Philip J. Landrigan, and Valerie M. Thomas, "Relation of Blood Lead Levels and Lead in Gasoline: An Updated Systematic Review," *Environmental Health* 21, no. 138 (2022). https://doi .org/10.1186/s12940-022-00936-x.

Bilefsky, Dan, and Jane Perlez, "Vaclav Havel, Former Czech President, Dies at 75," *New York Times*, December 11, 2011. https://www.nytimes.com /2011/12/19/world/europe/vaclav-havel-dissident-playwright-who-led -czechoslovakia-dead-at-75.html.

Centola, Damon, "Damon Centola" (home page). Accessed September 16, 2024, https://www.damoncentola.com/.

Clean Water Action, "Newark Makes History with First-in-the-Nation Environmental Justice Ordinance," 2024. Accessed September 16, 2024, https://cleanwater.org/newark-makes-history-first-nation-environmental -justice-ordinance.

Harley, Kim G., et al., "Reducing Phthalate, Paraben, and Phenol Exposure from Personal Care Products in Adolescent Girls: Findings from the HERMOSA Intervention Study," *Environmental Health Perspectives* 124, no. 10 (2016): 1600–1607. https://pubmed.ncbi.nlm.nih.gov/26947464/.

Hertz-Picciotto, Irva, et al., "Organophosphate Exposures During Pregnancy and Child Neurodevelopment: Recommendations for Essential Policy Reforms," *PLoS Medicine* 15, no. 10 (2018). https://doi.org/10.1371/journal.pmed .1002671.

Kaur, Rajwinder, et al., "Pesticides: An Alarming Detrimental to Health and Environment," *Science of the Total Environment* 915 (2024). https://doi.org /10.1016/j.scitotenv.2024.170113.

Liu, Jianghong, and Erin Schelar, "Pesticide Exposure and Child Neurodevelopment," *Workplace Health & Safety* 60, no. 5 (2014): 235–43. https://doi.org/10.1177/216507991206000507.

Pirkle, James L., et al., "The Decline in Blood Lead Levels in the United States: The National Health and Nutrition Examination Surveys (NHANES)," *Journal of the American Medical Association* 272, no. 4 (1994): 284–91. https://doi.org/10.1001/jama.1994.03520040046039.

Portela de-Assis, Mariana, et al., "Health Problems in Agricultural Workers Occupationally Exposed to Pesticides," *Revista Brasileira de Medicina do Trabalho* 18, no. 3 (2021): 352–63. https://doi.org/10.47626/1679-4435- 2020-532.

Rudel, Ruthann A., et al., "Food Packaging and Bisphenol A and Bis(2-Ethyhexyl) Phthalate Exposure: Findings from a Dietary Intervention," *Environmental Health Perspectives* 119, no. 7 (2011): 914–20. https://doi .org/10.1289/ehp.1003170.

Zota, Ami R., Antonia M. Calafat, and Tracey J. Woodruff, "Temporal Trends in Phthalate Exposures: Findings from the National Health and Nutrition Examination Survey, 2001–2010," *Environmental Health Perspectives* 122, no. 3 (2014): 235–41. https://doi.org/10.1289/ehp.1306681.

Alliance for Cancer Prevention, "The Prague Declaration on Endocrine Disruption," signed by Ronny Van Aerle et al., August 2005. https:// allianceforcancerprevention.org.uk/wp-content/uploads/2012/02/the -prague-declaration.pdf.

American College of Obstetricians and Gynecologists, "Reducing Prenatal Exposure to Toxic Environmental Agents," Committee Opinion no. 832, July 2021. https://www.acog.org/Clinical/Clinical-Guidance/Committee -Opinion/Articles/2021/07/Reducing-Prenatal-Exposure-to-Toxic -Environmental-Agents.

Collaborative for Health & Environment, "Vallombrosa Consensus Statement on Environmental Contaminants and Human Fertility Compromise," signed by Linda C. Giudice et al., October 2005. https://www.healthand environment.org/docs/xaruploads/VallombrosaConsensusStatement.pdf.

Demeneix, Barbara, Laura N. Vandenberg, Richard Ivel, and Thomas R. Zoeller, "Thresholds and Endocrine Disruptors: An Endocrine Society Policy Perspective," *Journal of the Endocrine Society* 4, no. 10 (2020). https://doi .org/10.1210/jendso/bvaa085.

Diamanti-Kandarakis, Evanthia, et al., "Endocrine-Disrupting Chemicals: An Endocrine Society Scientific Statement," *Endocrine Reviews* 30, no. 4 (2009): 293–342. https://doi.org/10.1210/er.2009-0002.

DiGangi, Joseph, et al., "San Antonio Statement on Brominated and Chlorinated Flame Retardants," *Environmental Health Perspectives* 118, no. 12 (December 2010). https://doi.org/10.1289/ehp.1003089.

Dréno, Brigitte, et al., "Safety Review of Phenoxyethanol When Used as a Preservative in Cosmetics," *Journal of the European Academy of Dermatology and Venereology* 33, no. 7 (2019): 15–24. https://doi.org/10.1111/jdv.15944.

Druckman, James N., et al., "Affective Polarization, Local Contexts, and Public Opinion in America," *Nature Human Behavior* 5 (2021): 28–38. https://doi .org/10.1038/s41562-020-01012-5.

Gore, Andrea C., et al., "EDC-2: The Endocrine Society's Second Scientific Statement on Endocrine-Disrupting Chemicals," *Endocrine Reviews* 36, no. 6 (2015): E1–150. https://doi.org/10.1210/er.2015-1010.

Haidt, Jonathan, *The Anxious Generation: How the Great Rewiring of Childhood Is Causing an Epidemic of Mental Illness.* Penguin Press (2024).

International Federation of Gynecology and Obstetrics, "FIGO Statement: FIGO Calls for Removal of PFAS from Global Use," May 25, 2021. https:// www.figo.org/figo-calls-removal-pfas-global-use.

International Federation of Gynecology and Obstetrics, "FIGO Statement: Toxic Chemicals and Environmental Contaminants in Prenatal Vitamins," 2023. https://www.figo.org/resources/figo-statements/toxic-chemicals-and -environmental-contaminants-prenatal-vitamins.

International Federation of Gynecology and Obstetrics, "Media Statement: Environmental Threats to Human Health," October 1, 2018. https://www .figo.org/Congress2018-Enviromental-Health.

International Programme on Chemical Safety, *Global Assessment on the State of the Science of Endocrine Disruptors,* World Health Organization (2002). https:// iris.who.int/handle/10665/67357.

Kahn, Linda G., et al., "Endocrine-Disrupting Chemicals: Implications for Human Health," *The Lancet: Diabetes & Endocrinology* 8, no. 8 (2020): 703–18. https://doi.org/10.1016/S2213-8587(20)30129-7.

Kassotis, Christopher D., et al., "Endocrine-Disrupting Chemicals: Economic, Regulatory, and Policy Implications," *The Lancet: Diabetes & Endocrinology* 8, no. 8 (2020): 719–30. https://doi.org/10.1016/S2213-8587(20)30128-5.

Kelm, Ole, et al., "How Algorithmically Curated Online Environments Influence Users' Political Polarization: Results from Two Experiments with Panel Data," *Computers in Human Behavior Reports* 12 (2023). https://doi .org/10.1016/j.chbr.2023.100343.

Korioth, Trisha, "Updated AAP Manual Addresses Pediatric Environmental Health Issues," American Academy of Pediatrics, May 2019. https:// publications.aap.org/aapnews/news/14573?autologincheck=redirected.

La Merrill, Michele A., et al., "Consensus on the Key Characteristics of Endocrine-Disrupting Chemicals as a Basis for Hazard Identification," *Nature Reviews Endocrinology* 16 (2020): 45–57. https://doi.org/10.1038 /s41574-019-0273-8.

National Institute of Environmental Health Sciences (NIEHS), National Toxicology Program, "Endocrine Disruptors Low-Dose Peer Review," October 2000. https://ntp.niehs.nih.gov/sites/default/files/ntp/pressctr /mtgs_wkshps/2000/lowdoseprogram.pdf.

National Research Council Committee on Hormonally Active Agents in the Environment, *Hormonally Active Agents in the Environment*. National Academies Press (1999). https://www.ncbi.nlm.nih.gov/books /NBK230233/.

Page, Jamie, et al., "A New Consensus on Reconciling Fire Safety with Environmental and Health Impacts of Chemical Flame Retardants," *Environment International* 173 (2023). https://doi.org/10.1016/j.envint .2023.107782.

Royal Society, "Endocrine Disrupting Chemicals (EDCs)," June 2000. https:// royalsociety.org/-/media/policy/publications/2000/10070.pdf.

Scientific Committee on Consumer Safety (SCCS), "Opinion on Phenoxyethanol," European Commission, October 6, 2016. https://health .ec.europa.eu/document/download/64bbaab3-66e2-44b8-817a-3d0e 313c3aaf_en.

SETAC Society, *Chemically Induced Alterations in Functional Development and Reproduction of Fishes*, edited by Michael Gilbertson, Richard E. Peterson, and Rosalind Rolland, proceedings of the Wingspread conference on "Chemically Induced Alterations in Functional Development and Reproduction of Fishes," Racine, Wisconsin, July 21–23, 1995 (SETAC Press, 1997). https://lib.ugent.be/catalog/rug01:001039616.

SETAC Society, "Chemically-Induced Alteration in Sexual Development: The Wildlife/Human Connection," conference at Wingspread Conference

Center, Racine, Wisconsin, July 1991. https://www.americanhealthstudies.org/wastenot/wn220.htm.

SETAC Society, "Statement from the Work Session on Chemically-Induced Alterations in the Developing Immune System: The Wildlife/Human Connection," *Environmental Health Perspectives* 104, no. 4 (1996): 807–8. https://ehp.niehs.nih.gov/doi/pdf/10.1289/ehp.104-1469664.

Solecki, Roland, et al., "Scientific Principles for the Identification of Endocrine-Disrupting Chemicals: A Consensus Statement," *Archives of Toxicology* 91, no. 2 (2017): 1001–6. https://doi.org/10.1007/s00204-016-1866-9.

"Statement from the Work Session on Environmental Endocrine-Disrupting Chemicals: Neural, Endocrine, and Behavioral Effects," consensus statement (the Erice Statement) from the conference held at International School of Ethology, Ettore Majorana Centre for Scientific Culture, Erice, Sicily, November 5–10, 1995, reprinted in *Toxicology and Industrial Health* 14, nos. 1/2 (1998). https://doi.org/10.1177/074823379801400103.

"Statement from the Work Session on Environmentally Induced Alterations in Development: A Focus on Wildlife," consensus statement from Wingspread Conference on "Environmentally Induced Alterations in Development: A Focus on Wildlife," Racine, Wisconsin, December 1995, reprinted in *Environmental Health Perspectives* 103, no. 4 (1995): 3–5. https://pmc.ncbi.nlm.nih.gov/articles/PMC1519268/.

Vos, Joseph G., et al., "Health Effects of Endocrine-Disrupting Chemicals on Wildlife, with Special Reference to the European Situation," *Critical Reviews in Toxicology* 30, no. 1 (2000): 71–133. https://doi.org/10.1080/10408440091159176.

ADDITIONAL RESOURCES

Alliance for Cancer Prevention, "The Prague Declaration on Endocrine Disruption," signed by Ronny Van Aerle et al., August 2005. https://alliance-forcancerprevention.org.uk/wp-content/uploads/2012/02/the-prague-declaration.pdf.

American College of Obstetricians and Gynecologists, "Reducing Prenatal Exposure to Toxic Environmental Agents," Committee Opinion no. 832, July 2021. https://www.acog.org/Clinical/Clinical-Guidance/Committee-Opinion/Articles/2021/07/Reducing-Prenatal-Exposure-to-Toxic-Environmental-Agents.

Collaborative for Health & Environment, "Vallombrosa Consensus Statement on Environmental Contaminants and Human Fertility Compromise," signed by Linda C. Giudice et al., October 2005. https://www.healthandenvironment.org/docs/xaruploads/VallombrosaConsensusStatement.pdf.

Demeneix, Barbara, Laura N. Vandenberg, Richard Ivel, and Thomas R. Zoeller, "Thresholds and Endocrine Disruptors: An Endocrine Society Policy Perspective," *Journal of the Endocrine Society* 4, no. 10 (2020). https://doi.org/10.1210/jendso/bvaa085.

Diamanti-Kandarakis, Evanthia, et al., "Endocrine-Disrupting Chemicals: An Endocrine Society Scientific Statement," *Endocrine Reviews* 30, no. 4 (2009): 293–342. https://doi.org/10.1210/er.2009-0002.

DiGangi, Joseph, et al., "San Antonio Statement on Brominated and Chlorinated Flame Retardants," *Environmental Health Perspectives* 118, no. 12 (December 2010). https://doi.org/10.1289/ehp.1003089.

Dréno, Brigitte, et al., "Safety Review of Phenoxyethanol When Used as a Preservative in Cosmetics," *Journal of the European Academy of Dermatology and Venereology* 33, no. 7 (2019): 15–24. https://doi.org/10.1111/jdv.15944.

Druckman, James N., et al., "Affective Polarization, Local Contexts, and Public Opinion in America," *Nature Human Behavior* 5 (2021): 28–38. https://doi.org/10.1038/s41562-020-01012-5.

Gore, Andrea C., et al., "EDC-2: The Endocrine Society's Second Scientific Statement on Endocrine-Disrupting Chemicals," *Endocrine Reviews* 36, no. 6 (2015): E1–150. https://doi.org/10.1210/er.2015-1010.

Haidt, Jonathan, *The Anxious Generation: How the Great Rewiring of Childhood Is Causing an Epidemic of Mental Illness*. Penguin Press (2024).

International Federation of Gynecology and Obstetrics, "FIGO Statement: FIGO Calls for Removal of PFAS from Global Use," May 25, 2021. https://www.figo.org/figo-calls-removal-pfas-global-use.

International Federation of Gynecology and Obstetrics, "FIGO Statement: Toxic Chemicals and Environmental Contaminants in Prenatal Vitamins," 2023. https://www.figo.org/resources/figo-statements/toxic-chemicals-and-environmental-contaminants-prenatal-vitamins.

International Federation of Gynecology and Obstetrics, "Media Statement: Environmental Threats to Human Health," October 1, 2018. https://www.figo.org/Congress2018-Enviromental-Health.

International Programme on Chemical Safety, *Global Assessment on the State of the Science of Endocrine Disruptors*, World Health Organization (2002). https://iris.who.int/handle/10665/67357.

Kahn, Linda G., et al., "Endocrine-Disrupting Chemicals: Implications for Human Health," *The Lancet: Diabetes & Endocrinology* 8, no. 8 (2020): 703–18. https://doi.org/10.1016/S2213-8587(20)30129-7.

Kassotis, Christopher D., et al., "Endocrine-Disrupting Chemicals: Economic, Regulatory, and Policy Implications," *The Lancet: Diabetes & Endocrinology* 8, no. 8 (2020): 719–30. https://doi.org/10.1016/S2213-8587(20)30128-5.

Kelm, Ole, et al., "How Algorithmically Curated Online Environments Influence Users' Political Polarization: Results from Two Experiments with Panel Data," *Computers in Human Behavior Reports* 12 (2023). https://doi.org/10.1016/j.chbr.2023.100343.

Korioth, Trisha, "Updated AAP Manual Addresses Pediatric Environmental Health Issues," American Academy of Pediatrics, May 2019. https://publications.aap.org/aapnews/news/14573?autologincheck=redirected.

La Merrill, Michele A., et al., "Consensus on the Key Characteristics of Endocrine-Disrupting Chemicals as a Basis for Hazard Identification," *Nature Reviews Endocrinology* 16 (2020): 45–57. https://doi.org/10.1038/s41574-019-0273-8.

National Institute of Environmental Health Sciences (NIEHS), National Toxicology Program, "Endocrine Disruptors Low-Dose Peer Review," October 2000. https://ntp.niehs.nih.gov/sites/default/files/ntp/pressctr/mtgs_wkshps/2000/lowdoseprogram.pdf.

National Research Council Committee on Hormonally Active Agents in the Environment, *Hormonally Active Agents in the Environment*. National Academies Press (1999). https://www.ncbi.nlm.nih.gov/books/NBK230233/.

Page, Jamie, et al., "A New Consensus on Reconciling Fire Safety with Environmental and Health Impacts of Chemical Flame Retardants," *Environment International* 173 (2023). https://doi.org/10.1016/j.envint.2023.107782.

Royal Society, "Endocrine Disrupting Chemicals (EDCs)," June 2000. https://royalsociety.org/-/media/policy/publications/2000/10070.pdf.

Scientific Committee on Consumer Safety (SCCS), "Opinion on Phenoxyethanol," European Commission, October 6, 2016. https://health.ec.europa.eu/document/download/64bbaab3-66e2-44b8-817a-3d0e313c3aaf_en.

SETAC Society, *Chemically Induced Alterations in Functional Development and Reproduction of Fishes*, edited by Michael Gilbertson, Richard E. Peterson, and Rosalind Rolland, proceedings of the Wingspread conference on "Chemically Induced Alterations in Functional Development and Reproduction of Fishes," Racine, Wisconsin, July 21–23, 1995 (SETAC Press, 1997). https://lib.ugent.be/catalog/rug01:001039616.

SETAC Society, "Chemically-Induced Alteration in Sexual Development: The Wildlife/Human Connection," conference at Wingspread Conference Center, Racine, Wisconsin, July 1991. https://www.americanhealthstudies.org/wastenot/wn220.htm.

SETAC Society, "Statement from the Work Session on Chemically-Induced Alterations in the Developing Immune System: The Wildlife/Human Connection," *Environmental Health Perspectives* 104, no. 4 (1996): 807–8. https://ehp.niehs.nih.gov/doi/pdf/10.1289/ehp.104-1469664.

Solecki, Roland, et al., "Scientific Principles for the Identification of Endocrine-Disrupting Chemicals: A Consensus Statement," *Archives of Toxicology* 91, no. 2 (2017): 1001–6. https://doi.org/10.1007/s00204 -016-1866-9.

"Statement from the Work Session on Environmental Endocrine-Disrupting Chemicals: Neural, Endocrine, and Behavioral Effects," consensus statement (the Erice Statement) from the conference held at International School of Ethology, Ettore Majorana Centre for Scientific Culture, Erice, Sicily, November 5–10, 1995, reprinted in *Toxicology and Industrial Health* 14, no. 1–2 (1998). https://doi.org/10.1177/074823379801400103.

"Statement from the Work Session on Environmentally Induced Alterations in Development: A Focus on Wildlife," consensus statement from Wingspread Conference on "Environmentally Induced Alterations in Development: A Focus on Wildlife," Racine, Wisconsin, December 1995, reprinted in *Environmental Health Perspectives* 103, no. 4 (1995): 3–5. https://pmc.ncbi.nlm.nih.gov/articles/PMC1519268/.

Vos, Joseph G., et al., "Health Effects of Endocrine-Disrupting Chemicals on Wildlife, with Special Reference to the European Situation," *Critical Reviews in Toxicology* 30, no. 1 (2000): 71–133. https://doi.org /10.1080/10408440091159176.

INDEX

Washington Post, 162
water bottles, 106
  BPA-free, 1–2, 9, 51
  polypropylene, 51, 231
  stainless steel, 2, 9, 122
water filters, 230
water supply. *See* drinking water
WE ACT for Environmental Justice, 216,
  220
web-savviness, 220
wellness industry, 130–31, 170–71
Wen Conditioner, 143

West Virginia, 92, 93, 97, 99, 100,
  101
Whac-a-Mole, 9, 38, 60
Whole Foods, 133
Wiig, Kristen, 144
Women's Voices for the Earth, 220
World War II, 83

Yuka (app), 207–8
Yupik peoples, 82–89

Zota, Ami, 159–61, 195–96, 222

ABOUT THE AUTHOR

Lindsay Dahl is a mom and activist who has helped pass over thirty state and federal laws that remove toxic chemicals from consumer products and the environment. A nationally awarded social impact leader, Dahl has been featured in the *New York Times*, *Fast Company*, and *Vogue*, among other publications. Dahl has worked across leadership positions for environmental health nonprofits, including Safer Chemicals, Healthy Families, and for leading clean consumer brands, including Ritual and Beautycounter. She sits on the board of directors for the nonprofits Toxic-Free Future and the Chamber of Mothers.

To view Lindsay's brand recommendations, visit heyhilde.com